GABA AND BENZODIAZEPINE RECEPTOR SUBTYPES
Molecular Biology, Pharmacology, and Clinical Aspects

Advances in Biochemical Psychopharmacology
Volume 46

Advances in Biochemical Psychopharmacology

Series Editors

E. Costa, M.D.

Director
Fidia-Georgetown Institute for the Neurosciences
Georgetown University Medical Center
Washington, DC 20007

Paul Greengard, Ph.D.

Professor of Molecular and Cellular Neuroscience
The Rockefeller University
1230 York Avenue
New York, NY 10021

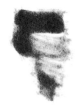

GABA and Benzodiazepine Receptor Subtypes

Molecular Biology, Pharmacology, and Clinical Aspects

Advances in Biochemical Psychopharmacology
Volume 46

Volume Editors

Giovanni Biggio, Ph.D.
*Department of Experimental
  Biology
University of Cagliari
Cagliari, Italy*

Erminio Costa, M.D.
*Fidia-Georgetown Institute for
  the Neurosciences
Georgetown University Medical
  Center
Washington, DC*

Raven Press *New York*

Raven Press, 1185 Avenue of the Americas, New York, New York 10036

Made in the United States of America

Library of Congress Cataloging-in-Publication Data

GABA and benzodiazepine receptor subtypes : molecular biology, pharmacology, and clinical aspects / volume editors, Giovanni Biggio, Erminio Costa.
    p. cm. — (Advances in biochemical psychopharmacology ; v. 46)
    The proceedings of the 6th Capo Boi Conference on Neuroscience held at Villasimius, Italy, in June 1989.
    Includes bibliographical references.
    Includes index.
    ISBN 0-88167-697-7
    1. GABA—Receptors—Congresses. 2. Benzodiazepines—Receptors-
-Congresses. I.Biggio, Giovanni. II. Costa, Erminio.
III. Series.
    [DNLM: 1. Receptors, GABA-Benzodiazepine—isolation &
purification—congresses. 2. Receptors, GABA-Benzodiazepine-
-pharmacology—congresses. W1 AD437 v. 46 / WK 102 G112 1989]
RM315.A4 vol. 46
[QP364.7]
615′.78 s—dc20
[599′.0188]
DNLM/DLC
for Library of Congress   90-8829
                                                CIP

9 8 7 6 5 4 3 2 1

Preface

The progress in our understanding of the GABAergic synaptic function has contributed a structural complexity that five years ago would have been unthinkable. Now this puzzle is in front of us for interpretation. Indeed, it is not easy to assess whether or not all the possible combinations of the $GABA_A$ receptor subtypes (more than 10^4) are expressed and functional. Moreover, the myth that the benzodiazepine recognition sites would be linked exclusively to the GABAergic function has vanished with the cloning of mitochondrial recognition sites located in the outer membrane of a selected population of mitochondria. However, these receptors can be linked to the GABAergic function only indirectly and, perhaps, not exclusively. In fact, it is becoming clear that the recognition site for the peripheral benzodiapines may be associated with the cholesterol transport across the outer mitochondrial membrane and linked to steroidogenesis. It is now emerging that one or more steroid derivatives probably synthesized in glial cells may function in the modulation of GABAergic transmission at a site located in the proximity of the gating mechanism regulating the anionic channels operated by GABA. The mitochondrial recognition site for benzodiazepines is not uniformly distributed in every mitochondrial membrane of various tissues (it appears to be more abundant in adrenal cortex and testicles), and it may be specifically located in some cells of various organs (Leydig's cells, testicles, and glial cells in brain). The possibility that specific steroids produced in glial cells are associated with the function of GABA receptors has become an attractive working hypothesis. An answer to this question may allow some interesting speculation about the etiology of anxiety disorders.

The structural diversity of the α subunit where the benzodiazepine recognition site appears to be located opens the possibility that specific classes of benzodiazepines may exist that preferentially or exclusively act on specific $GABA_A$ receptor subtypes. Hence, it is hoped that classes of benzodiazepines can be singled out for their capability to ameliorate the synthomatology of selected groups of anxiety disorders. It is also becoming clear that, though the benzodiazepine recognition site is located in the α subunit, the γ subunit is an essential requirement for the expression of the positive (benzodiazepines) or negative (betacarbolines) modulation of $GABA_A$ receptors. The molecular mechanism whereby γ_1 and γ_2 subunits interact with the α subunits is not yet understood. However, it is known that the diversity of the γ subunits (γ_1 and γ_2) not only exerts a permissive action on the allosteric modulation of the GABA recognition site of $GABA_A$ receptors but also determines the direction of the modulatory action of various ligands.

The endogenous peptides acting as ligands for the central and peripheral benzodiazepine recognition sites derive from the propeptide DBI (diazepam binding inhibitor). Now they are better understood in terms of the specificity of their biological action. The DBI cloning has been obtained by various research teams working on different biological problems. Thus, endocrinologists have suggested that DBI or its processing products may be operative in mediating the mitochondrial steroidogenesis of the pituitary gonadotropic hormones by binding to the peripheral recognition sites for the benzodiapines of mitochondria. Biochemists have suggested that DBI is operative in the regulation of lipid chain elongation where it appears to mediate the action of CoA. In the neurosciences the study of DBI and its processing products as putative endogenous modulators of the affinity of GABA recognition site on $GABA_A$ receptors continues. The DBI processing in various cell types is actively investigated and the possible existence of more than one mRNA encoding for DBI is studied.

The findings reported here may even allow a greater number of inferences that have not been delineated in this speculative preface. One must wait for pertinent findings to consolidate or destroy some of these speculations. Future research may generate alternative working hypotheses without validating or destroying the present speculations. This volume will be of interest to neuroscientists, pharmacologists, cell biologists, molecular biologists, and neurologists.

Contents

Acknowledgments

This volume presents the proceedings of the 6th Capo Boi Conference on Neuroscience held at Villasimius, Italy, in June 1989. This Conference was realized by the generous support given by the Fidia Research Laboratories of Abano Terme, Italy. The Editors would like to take this opportunity to express their gratitude and appreciation.

Contributors

Lucyna Antkiewicz-Michaluk
Fidia-Georgetown Institute for the
* Neurosciences*
Georgetown University School of
* Medicine*
3900 Reservoir Road, N.W.
Washington, D.C. 20007

M. D. Antonacci
Fidia-Georgetown Institute for the
* Neurosciences*
Georgetown University School of
* Medicine*
Suite SE-402
3900 Reservoir Road, N.W.
Washington, D.C. 20007

S. Arbilla
Department of Biology
Synthélabo Recherche (L.E.R.S.)
58, rue de la Glacière
75013 Paris, France

M. Baraldi
Cattedra di Farmacologia e
* Farmacognosia della Facoltà di*
* Farmacia*
Università di Modena
41100 Modena, Italy

Anthony S. Basile
Section on Neurobiology
Laboratory of Neuroscience,
* NIDDK*
National Institutes of Health
Bethesda, Maryland 20892

J. Benavides
Department of Biology
Synthélabo Recherche (L.E.R.S.)
58, rue de la Glacière
75013 Paris, France

A. Berkovich
Fidia-Georgetown Institute for the
* Neurosciences*
Georgetown University School of
* Medicine*
3900 Reservoir Road, N.W.
Washington, D.C. 20007

Giovanni Biggio
Department of Experimental
* Biology*
University of Cagliari
09100 Cagliari, Italy

G. Bovolin
Fidia-Georgetown Institute for the
* Neurosciences*
Georgetown University School of
* Medicine*
3900 Reservoir Road, N.W.
Washington, D.C. 20007

N. G. Bowery
Department of Pharmacology
The School of Pharmacy
29/39 Brunswick Square
WC1N 1AX London, England

N. Brecha
Department of Anatomy
Brain Research Institute
University of California
Los Angeles, California 90024

M. Bureau
Department of Pharmacology
Brain Research Institute
University of California
Los Angeles, California 90024

G. B. Cassano
Department of Psychiatry
via Rome 67
University of Pisa
56100 Pisa, Italy

M.-Y. Chiang
Department of Biology
Brain Research Institute
University of California
Los Angeles, California 90024

A. Concas
Department of Experimental
Biology
Chair of Pharmacology
University of Cagliari
Cagliari, Italy

M.G. Corda
Department of Experimental
Biology
Chair of Pharmacology
University of Cagliari
Cagliari, Italy

E. Costa
Fidia-Georgetown Institute for the
Neurosciences
Georgetown University School of
Medicine
3900 Reservoir Road, N.W.
Washington, D.C. 20007

A. Draguhn
Max-Planck-Institut für
Medizinische Forschung
Heidelberg, FRG

Sergio H. Gammal
Liver Diseases Section
Digestive Diseases Branch, NIDDK
National Institutes of Health
Bethesda, Maryland 20892

G. Giannaccini
"Istituto Policattedra di Discipline
Biologiche"
via Bonanno 6
University of Pisa
56100 Pisa, Italy

O. Giorgi
Department of Experimental
Biology
Chair of Pharmacology
University of Cagliari
Cagliari, Italy

P. Giusti
Fidia-Georgetown Institute for the
Neurosciences
Georgetown University School of
Medicine
Suite SE-402
3900 Reservoir Road, N.W.
Washington, D.C. 20007

Dennis R. Grayson
Fidia-Georgetown Institute for the
  Neurosciences
Georgetown University School of
  Medicine
3900 Reservoir Road, N.W.
Washington, D.C. 20007

David J. Greenblatt
Division of Clinical Pharmacology
Departments of Psychiatry and
  Pharmacology
Tufts University School of
  Medicine
New England Medical Center
Boston, Massachusetts 02111

P. Guarneri
Fidia-Georgetown Institute for the
  Neurosciences
Georgetown University School of
  Medicine
3900 Reservoir Road, N.W.
Washington, D.C. 20007

Alessandro Guidotti
Fidia-Georgetown Institute for the
  Neurosciences
Georgetown University School of
  Medicine
3900 Reservoir Road, N.W.
Washington, D.C. 20007

Willy Haefely
Pharmaceutical Research
  Department
F. Hoffmann-LaRoche Ltd.
CH-4002 Basel, Switzerland

Jack Heller
Division of Clinical Pharmacology
Departments of Psychiatry and
  Pharmacology
Tufts University School of
  Medicine
New England Medical Center
Boston, Massachusetts 02111

M. Jackson
Department of Biology
Brain Research Institute
University of California
Los Angeles, California 90024

E. Anthony Jones
Liver Diseases Section
Digestive Diseases Branch, NIDDK
National Institutes of Health
Bethesda, Maryland 20892

G. L. Kamatchi
Department of Pharmacology
The University of Texas Health
  Science Center at San Antonio
7703 Floyd Curl Drive
San Antonio, Texas 78284-7764

M. Khrestchatisky
Department of Biology
Brain Research Institute
University of California
Los Angeles, California 90024

C. Knott
Department of Pharmacology
The School of Pharmacy
29/39 Brunswick Square
WC1N 1AX London, England

Karl E. Krueger
Fidia-Georgetown Institute for the
  Neurosciences
Georgetown University School of
  Medicine
3900 Reservoir Road, N.W.
Washington, D.C. 20007

S. Z. Langer
Synthélabo Recherche (L.E.R.S.)
58, rue de la Glacière
75013 Paris, France

B. Longoni
Department of Experimental
  Biology
Chair of Pharmacology
University of Cagliari
Cagliari, Italy

Fred Lopez
Division of Clinical Pharmacology
Departments of Psychiatry and
  Pharmacology
Tufts University School of
  Medicine
New England Medical Center
Boston, Massachusetts 02111

A. Lucacchini
"Istituto Policattedra di Discipline
  Biologiche"
via Bonanno 6
University of Pisa
56100 Pisa, Italy

Monica Lumpkin
Division of Clinical Pharmacology
Departments of Psychiatry and
  Pharmacology
Tufts University School of
  Medicine
New England Medical Center
Boston, Massachusetts 02111

A. J. MacLennan
Department of Biology
Brain Research Institute
University of California
Los Angeles, California 90024

P. Malherbe
Pharmaceutical Research
  Department
F. Hoffmann-LaRoche Ltd.
Basel, Italy

D. Marazziti
Department of Psychiatry
via Rome 67
University of Pisa
56100 Pisa, Italy

C. Martini
"Istituto Policattedra di Discipline
  Biologiche"
via Bonanno 6
University of Pisa
56100 Pisa, Italy
"Istituto di Chimica Biologica"
University of Parma
43100 Parma, Italy

M. P. Mascia
Department of Experimental
  Biology
Chair of Pharmacology
University of Cagliari
Cagliari, Italy

M. Massotti
Laboratorio di Farmacologia
Istituto Superiore di Sanita
00161 Roma, Italy

A. K. Mehta
Department of Pharmacology
The University of Texas Health
  Science Center at San Antonio
7703 Floyd Curl Drive
San Antonio, Texas 78284-7764

M. Memo
Fidia-Georgetown Institute for the
  Neurosciences
Georgetown University School of
  Medicine
Suite SE-402
3900 Reservoir Road, N.W.
Washington, D.C. 20007

Giampaolo Mereu
Department of Experimental
  Biology
"Bernardo Loddo" Section of
  Neuroscience
University of Cagliari
09100 Cagliari, Italy

S. Michelini
Department of Psychiatry
via Rome 67
University of Pisa
56100 Pisa, Italy

Lawrence G. Miller
Division of Clinical Pharmacology
Departments of Psychiatry and
  Pharmacology
Tufts University School of
  Medicine
New England Medical Center
Boston, Massachusetts 02111

H. Mohler
Institute of Pharmacology
University of Zürich
Switzerland

R. Moratalla
Department of Pharmacology
The School of Pharmacy
29/39 Brunswick Square
WC1N 1AX London, England

Alexey G. Mukhin
Fidia-Georgetown Institute for the
  Neurosciences
Georgetown University School of
  Medicine
3900 Reservoir Road, N.W.
Washington, D.C. 20007

R. W. Olsen
Department of Pharmacology
Brain Research Institute
University of California
Los Angeles, California 90024

M. Orlandi
Department of Experimental
  Biology
Chair of Pharmacology
University of Cagliari
Cagliari, Italy

Nancy L. Ostrowski
Section on Clinical Brain Imaging
Laboratory on Cerebral
  Metabolism, NIMH
National Institutes of Health
Bethesda, Maryland 20892

E. Persohn
Pharmaceutical Research
  Department
F. Hoffmann-LaRoche Ltd.
Basel, Switzerland

G. D. Pratt
The School of Pharmacy
29/39 Brunswick Square
WC1N 1AX London, England

J. G. Richards
*Pharmaceutical Research
  Department
F. Hoffmann-LaRoche Ltd.
Basel, Switzerland*

E. Sanna
*Department of Experimental
  Biology
Chair of Pharmacology
University of Cagliari
Cagliari, Italy*

M. Rita Santi
*Fidia-Georgetown Institute for the
  Neurosciences
Georgetown University School of
  Medicine
3900 Reservoir Road, N.W.
Washington, D.C. 20007*

V. Santoro
*Department of Experimental
  Biology
Chair of Pharmacology
University of Cagliari
Cagliari, Italy*

B. Scatton
*Department of Biology
Synthélabo Recherche (L.E.R.S.)
58, rue de la Glacière
75013 Paris, France*

Andrew Schatzki
*Division of Clinical Pharmacology
Departments of Psychiatry and
  Pharmacology
Tufts University School of
  Medicine
New England Medical Center
Boston, Massachusetts 02111*

J. L. Schlichting
*Fidia-Georgetown Institute for the
  Neurosciences
Georgetown University School of
  Medicine
Suite SE-402
3900 Reservoir Road, N.W.
Washington, D.C. 20007*

Peter H. Seeburg
*Laboratory of Molecular
  Neuroendocrinology
Zentrum für Molekulare Biologie
University of Heidelberg
Im Neuenheimer Feld 282
6900 Heidelberg, FRG*

J. M. Sequier
*Pharmaceutical Research
  Department
F. Hoffmann-LaRoche Ltd.
Basel, Switzerland*

M. Serra
*Department of Experimental
  Biology
Chair of Pharmacology
University of Cagliari
Cagliari, Italy*

Richard I. Shader
*Division of Clinical Pharmacology
Departments of Psychiatry and
  Pharmacology
Tufts University School of
  Medicine
New England Medical Center
Boston, Massachusetts 02111*

E. Sigel
*Institute of Pharmacology
University of Bern
Bern, Switzerland*

Phil Skolnick
Section of Neurobiology
Laboratory of Neurosciences,
NIDDK
National Institutes of Health
Bethesda, Maryland 20892

E. Slobodyansky
Fidia-Georgetown Institute for the
Neurosciences
Georgetown University School of
Medicine
3900 Reservoir Road, N.W.
Washington, D.C. 20007

Rolf Sprengel
Laboratory of Molecular
Neuroendocrinology
Zentrum für Molekulare Biologie
University of Heidelberg
6900 Heidelberg, FRG

C. Sternini
Department of Medicine
Brain Research Institute
University of California
Los Angeles, California 90024

M. K. Ticku
Department of Pharmacology
The University of Texas Health
Science Center at San Antonio
7703 Floyd Curl Drive
San Antonio, Texas 78284-7764

A.J. Tobin
Department of Biology
Brain Research Institute
University of California
Los Angeles, California 90024

C. Wambebe
Fidia-Georgetown Institute for the
Neurosciences
Georgetown University School of
Medicine
3900 Reservoir Road, N.W.
Washington, D.C. 20007

Pia Werner
Laboratory of Molecular
Neuroendocrinology
Zentrum für Molekular Biologie
University of Heidelberg
6900 Heidelberg, FRG

W. Xu
Department of Biology
Brain Research Institute
University of California
Los Angeles, California 90024

P. Zanoli
Cattedra di Farmacologia e
Farmacognosia della Facoltà di
Farmacia
Università di Modena
41100 Modena, Italy

M. L. Zeneroli
Dipartimento di Scienze
Farmaceutiche e Cattedra di
Semeiotica Medica della Facoltà
di Medicina
Università di Modena
41100 Modena, Italy

GABA and Benzodiazepine Receptor Subtypes,
edited by Giovanni Biggio and Erminio Costa.
Raven Press, New York © 1990.

PURIFICATION, CLONING, AND EXPRESSION OF A
PERIPHERAL-TYPE BENZODIAZEPINE RECEPTOR

Karl E. Krueger, Alexey G. Mukhin, Lucyna Antkiewicz-Michaluk,
M. Rita Santi, Dennis R. Grayson, and Alessandro Guidotti

Fidia-Georgetown Institute for the Neurosciences
Georgetown University Medical School
Washington, D.C. 20007 U.S.A.

and

Rolf Sprengel, Pia Werner, and Peter H. Seeburg

Laboratory of Molecular Neuroendocrinology
Zentrum für Molekulare Biologie
University of Heidelberg
6900 Heidelberg, FRG

Ever since the initial discovery of specific binding sites
in the brain for benzodiazepines it had been demonstrated that
another class of binding sites for this group of drugs exists
in peripheral tissues (6). While the control pharmacological
actions of benzodiazepines are clearly mediated through their
binding to $GABA_A$-coupled chloride channels (7,8,28), the
possible pharmacological actions related to benzodiazepines
binding to the peripheral-type benzodiazepine recognition sites
(PBR) are not known. In order to understand the function of
PBR a detailed characterization of the molecular components of
these sites is essential.

PBR, in addition to being abundant in many peripheral
tissues, were also distinguished from $GABA_A$/benzodiazepine
receptors due to their differing binding specificity (24,34)
and subcellular localization. PBR are found primarily
associated with the mitochondrial compartment (1,2), although
other evidence suggests they may be located on other organelles
as well (10,26). While $GABA_A$ receptors are abundant in
neuronal cells, within the central nervous system PBR are most
prevalent in glial cells (14). In addition to binding various
benzodiazepine derivatives, PBR recognize a very wide array of

different organic compounds including isoquinoline carboxamides (22), quinoline propanamides (12), imidazopyridines (21), porphyrins (33), thiazide diuretics (23), and many others (16).

Some of the first attempts to begin a molecular characterization of PBR involved radiation inactivation studies. The target size estimated for the binding site of the PBR benzodiazepine ligand Ro5-4864 was 34 kDa (27) while the size determined for isoquinoline derivative PK 11195 was about 23 kDa (10). Since it had been demonstrated that the binding domains for benzodiazepines and isoquinoline carboxamides on PBR are not equivalent (5,30) this might indicate that separate proteins comprise the two recognition sites. The radiation inactivation studies were conducted by two different laboratories, therefore a direct comparison of their results may be misleading in interpreting whether a single or two separate proteins comprise these binding domains.

A number of affinity-labeling probes have been utilized in efforts to identify proteins associated with PBR. The benzodiazepine flunitrazepam was reported to photolabel proteins of 30-35 kDa in kidney mitochondrial preparations (31). Another benzodiazepine derivative, AHN 086, has also been recently reported to acylate a protein of 30 kDa from membrane preparations of the pineal gland (25). In contrast, PK 14105, an isoquinoline carboxamide photoaffinity probe, covalently modifies a 17-kDa protein (11). These studies therefore suggest that the binding domains for benzodiazepines and isoquinoline carboxamides reside on different proteins, although direct association of these identified proteins with PBR remains to be established.

Extensive evidence has been presented to demonstrate that PK 14105 specifically modifies PBR (11). Other isoquinoline carboxamides or benzodiazepines which show high affinities for PBR prevent photolabeling with [3H]PK 14105, while the photoincorporation is not blocked by benzodiazepines which show great selectivity for $GABA_A$ receptors. Furthermore, photolabeling of PBR with PK 14105 results in an irreversible inhibition of isoquinoline carboxamide and benzodiazepine binding. These observations provide strong evidence that PK 14105 specifically binds to and covalently modifies PBR at or near the recognition site for isoquinoline carboxamides.

These important findings prompted us to purify the 17-kDa protein photolabeled by PK 14105 and investigate its relationship to PBR. Included in this report is a description of the purification of this 17-kDa protein (entitled PKBS for PK binding site) and subsequent studies highlight the cloning and expression of the corresponding cDNA. These studies present evidence that expression of PKBS is required for the manifestation of PBR and that it apparently comprises the binding domains for benzodiazepines and for isoquinoline carboxamides.

RESULTS

Purification and partial amino acid sequencing of PKBS.

Since rat adrenal mitochondrial preparations possess a very high density of PBR, approximately 140 pmol/mg protein (2), this source was chosen to purify the 17-kDa PKBS protein. Based on the abundance of PBR in these membrane preparations PKBS is expected to comprise at least 0.2% of the total protein. The paradigm developed to subfractionate and monitor the purification of PKBS (3) involved combining rat adrenal mitochondrial membranes photolabeled with [^{3}H]PK 14105 with a 30-fold excess of unlabeled mitochondria. The membranes were then solubilized in a buffer containing 1% digitonin and proteins were fractionated by anion-exchange chromatography and reversed-phase high-pressure liquid chromatography. Table 1 lists representative recoveries of protein and radioactivity achieved throughout this scheme.

TABLE 1

Fraction	Total Protein (mg)	Total cpm (x 10^{-3})
Mitochondrial Membrane Fraction	90	1059
Digitonin-Solubilized Extract	82	903
Q-Sepharose	5.9	229
Reversed-Phase HPLC	0.12	40.0

Purified preparations obtained by this procedure exhibit a single protein species when electrophoresed and visualized by silver-staining or by radioiodination with Bolton-Hunter reagent (Fig. 1). In addition, this protein is covalently labeled with [^{3}H]PK 14105 and has the same size of 17 kDa as the [^{3}H]PK 14105 photolabeled adduct identified in intact mitochondria. As evaluated by these criteria PKBS has been purified to apparent homogeneity.

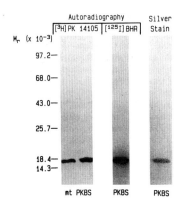

FIGURE 1

Electrophoretic analysis of purified PKBS. Samples
containing purified PKBS (1 μg protein, 2 x 10^3
cpm) or adrenal mitochondrial membranes (*mt*; 10
μg protein, 2 x 10^3 cpm) photolabeled with [^{3}H]PK
14105, or radioiodinated PKBS (1 x 10^5 cpm) were
electrophoresed on a 10-15% gradient polyacrylamide gel
(20). One portion of the gel was electroblotted to
nitrocellulose, the membrane sprayed with a flouro-
graphic enhancer, and autoradiographed. The section of
membrane containing sample radiolabeled with Bolton-
Hunter reagent ($[^{125}I]BHR$) was autoradiographed
separately with an intensifying screen. The remaining
portion of the gel was silver-stained.

For the purpose of cloning a cDNA for PKBS partial amino
sequences from the the purified protein were first determined.
When 200 pmol of purified PKBS was subjected to Edman
degradation it failed to produce phenylthiohydantoin
derivatives indicating that it is blocked at the amino
terminus. Hydrolysis of PKBS with cyanogen bromide and
subsequent chromatography of the digest over a C_{18} column
yielded five different peptide fragments which were partially
sequenced (Fig. 2). The amino acid sequences obtained
accounted for 86 residues, approximately one-half of the PKBS
polypeptide.

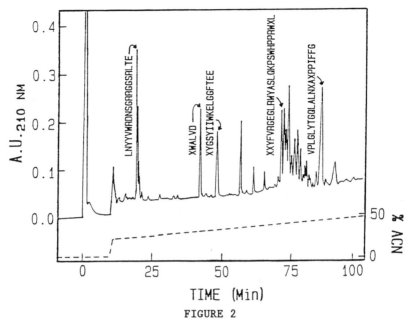

FIGURE 2

Isolation of PKBS peptide fragments. To a Vydac 201 TP reverse phase C_{18} column equilibrated in 0.1% tri-flouroacetic acid a cyanogen bromide digest (in 1.0 ml of 0.1% TFA), produced from approximately 100 μg of purified PKBS, was injected. After 6 min a single step-wise elution of 20% acetonitrile was performed followed by a linear gradient to 70% acetonitrile as shown in the lower section of the figure. Peptides which were isolated and subjected to gas-phase sequencing are indicated with their corresponding sequences. An *X* is represented where specific residue identification could not be made. *A.U.*, absorbance unit.

Cloning and sequencing of rat PKBS cDNA.

A rat adrenal cDNA library constructed in λgt10 was screened with two oligonucleotide probes whose sequences were based on the peptide sequence information. Of 1 x 10^6 recombinant plaques about 200 were identified by hybridization to both oligonucleotides and eight of these were analyzed further. All eight clones showed overlapping sequences among which the longest cDNA clone had an insert size of 781 base pairs. This included an open reading frame encoding a polypeptide of 169 amino acids (Fig. 3) which contains all peptide sequences from the isolated CNBr fragments of PKBS.

```
                                                  1                        10
                                          Met Ser Gln Ser Trp Val Pro Ala Val Gly Leu Thr
                  1 TGTGGATCTTTCCAGAACAGCAGTTGCAATCACT ATG TCT CAA TCC TGG GTA CCC GCC GTG GGC CTC ACT 70

---------------TM1-----------------
                  20                                    30                        40
Leu Val Pro Ser Leu Gly Gly Phe Met Gly Ala Tyr Phe Val Arg Gly Glu Gly Leu Arg Trp Tyr Ala Ser Leu Gln Lys Pro Ser Trp
CTG GTG CCG GCC CTG GGG GGC TTC ATG GGA GCC TAC TTT GTG CGT GGT GAG GGC CTC CGC TGG TAT GCT AGC TTG CAG AAA CCC TCC TGG 160

                                                      -TM2-
                  50                                    60                        70
His Pro Pro Arg Trp Thr Leu Ala Pro Ile Trp Gly Thr Leu Tyr Ser Ala Met Gly Tyr Gly Ser Tyr Ile Ile Trp Lys Glu Leu Gly
CAT CCG CCT CGC TGG ACA CTC GCT CCG ATC TGG GGC ACA CTG TAT TCG GCC ATG GGG TAT GGC TCC TAC ATA ATC TGG AAA GAG CTG GGA 250

                                                    -TM3-
                  80                                    90                       100
Gly Phe Thr Glu Glu Ala Met Val Pro Leu Gly Leu Tyr Thr Gly Gln Leu Ala Leu Asn Trp Ala Trp Pro Pro Ile Phe Phe Gly Ala
GGT TTC ACA GAG GAG GCT ATG GTT CCC TTG GGT CTC TAC ACT GGT CAG CTG GCT CTG AAC TGG GCA TGG CCC ATC TTC TTT GGT GCC 340

                                          -TM4-
                  110                                   120                      130
Arg Gln Met Gly Trp Ala Leu Val Asp Leu Met Leu Val Ser Gly Val Ala Thr Ala Thr Thr Leu Ala Trp His Arg Val Ser Pro Pro
CGG CAG ATG GGC TGG GCT TTG GTG GAC CTC ATG CTT GTC AGT GGG GTG GCA ACC GCC ACT ACC CTG GCT TGG CAC GGA GTG AGC CCA CCG 430

                                          -TM5-
                  140                                   150                      160
Ala Ala Arg Leu Leu Tyr Pro Tyr Leu Ala Trp Leu Ala Phe Ala Thr Met Leu Asn Tyr Tyr Val Trp Arg Asp Asn Ser Gly Arg Arg
GCT GCC GGC TTG CTG TAT CGT TAC CTG GCC TGG CTG GCC TTT GCC ACC ATG CTC AAC TAC TAT GTA TGG CGT GAT AAC TCT GGT CGG CGA 520

                  169
Gly Gly Ser Arg Leu Thr Glu
GGG GGC TCC CGG CTC ACA GAG TGA GGACACGTAGCCATCAGGAATGCAGGCGCTGGCAGCCAGGCATCATGGGTTGAGGTCATCCTGGCTTTCATGACCATTGGGCCTGCTGG 631

TCTACCTGGTCGTTAGTCCAGGAAGCCACCAGGTAGGTCAAGGTGGTCAGTGGTAAGTCGCATGCGGGGACAGTTGTACGTGCTTTTGTGCACAGCTGCAGGCGTGCCCTAGGAGCATGGG 751

GCCTTTAAAGGTAAATAAAGTGTTTAAGTT 781
```

FIGURE 3

Nucleotide and deduced amino acid sequence of the PKBS cDNA. The nucleotide sequence starting from the 5' end of the sense strand and the corresponding deduced amino acid sequence of the open reading frame are detailed. Potential transmembrane-spanning segments (TM1-TM5), as determined by the method of Eisenberg *et al.* (13), are indicated with brackets and the polyadenylation signal is underlined.

From the deduced amino acid sequence the primary translation product of PKBS is predicted to be 18,943 Da and to have an isoelectric point of about 9.1. Hydropathy analysis revealed a highly hydrophobic peptide profile with five potential transmembrane segments, referred to as TM1-TM5 (Figs. 3 and 4), which may account for the tight membrane association of PKBS.

A search for related proteins showed no significant similarity to any protein from several databases. Over 10 proteins, apparently unrelated to each other, showed similarity with PKBS to the extent of 30-45% identity within a 25 amino acid overlap, however. Among these similarities it was noticed that transmembrane-spanning segments M1, M2, and M4 from subunits of the GABA$_A$/benzodiazepine receptor family (28,29) show similarity with the sequences of seqments TM1, TM4, and TM5 from PKBS, respectively. Sequence identity relative to the

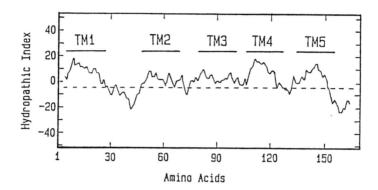

FIGURE 4

<u>Hydropathy analysis of PKBS.</u> Hydrophobicity profile
for the PKBS polypeptide sequence is shown as computed
using a window of nine amino acids (18,19).

PKBS sequence in these regions ranged from 18 to 41% while
conservative amino acid substitutions accounted for a 41-59%
degree of similarity. Nevertheless, since other proteins also
exhibit comparable degrees of similarity with PKBS, the
similarity with the GABA$_A$ receptor may only be coincidental.

<u>Expression of the PKBS cDNA in eukaryotic cells.</u>

The PKBS cDNA was inserted into an eukaryotic expression
pSV-globin plasmid (9,15) placing it under transcriptional
control of the β-globin promoter and the SV40 enhancer.
The transformed embryonal human kidney 293 cell line was used
for expression studies because these cells contain relatively
low levels of specific binding sites for the PBR ligands
Ro5-4864 and PK 11195 and serve as a suitable host for
transfection with the pSV-globin expression vector.

Single classes of specific binding sites for Ro5-4864 and PK
11195 were detected in 293 cells having dissociation constants
of 19 nM and 54 nM, respectively (Fig. 5). The relatively low
affinity observed for Ro5-4864 is characteristic of the
species-dependent differences previously reported in the
binding for this benzodiazepine (4,31,32).

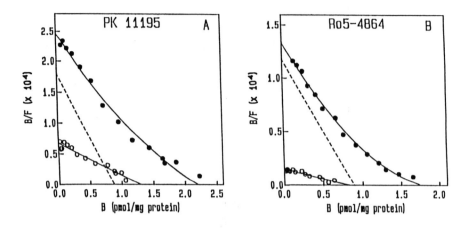

FIGURE 5

Scatchard analysis of [³H]PK 11195 and [³H]Ro5-4864 binding in transfected 293 cells. A representative experiment is shown where cell homogenates were examined for binding of (A) [³H]PK 11195 (0.3-155 nM) and (B) [³H]Ro5-4864 (1.3-200 nM). Nonspecific binding was determined in the presence of 10 μM of the corresponding nonradioactive ligand. Specific binding of the radioligands to mock-transfected 293 cells (O) and cells transfected with the pSV-PKBS vector (●) are shown as the mean of triplicate determinations. Computer-assisted nonlinear regression analysis using two-site models on data obtained with transfected cells was used to estimate the contributions of the higher affinity components by assuming that the lower affinity components were due to contribution of PBR also found in mock-transfected cells. *Broken lines* represent the higher affinity components resolved by this method. *Curves* drawn for the transfected cells are plotted based on these two-site models.

When the cells were transfected with the pSV-PKBS vector Scatchard analysis of Ro5-4864 and PK 11195 binding revealed an apparent biphasic relationship with concommitant increases of nearly 1 pmol/mg of protein in the B_{max} for both ligands. The lower affinity components appear to be equivalent to the single classes of binding sites observed in the mock-transfected 293 cells and therefore probably represent the endogenous human form of PBR expressed by 293 cells. The higher affinity components therefore are binding sites expressed following transfection with the pSV-PKBS vector. In contrast, cells transfected with either the parental pSV-globin plasmid, or a pSV plasmid carrying the PKBS cDNA in the opposite orientation, showed no differences in comparison with mock-transfected cells in PBR ligand binding characteristics (data not shown).

Nonlinear regression analysis performed on the binding data of pSV-PKBS transfected cells resolved higher affinity components having dissociation constants of 4.9 and 7.6 nM with B_{max} values of 880 and 890 fmol/mg of protein for PK 11195 and Ro5-4864, respectively (Fig. 5). It is noteworthy that the affinity observed for Ro5-4864 expressed following transfection with the rat PKBS expression vector is characteristic of rat PBR as opposed to the properties reported for PBR of human tissues.

To examine whether the expressed binding sites exhibit the same binding specificity as PBR normally found in rat tissues the potencies of different ligands in competing for [^{3}H]Ro5-4864 binding were tested. These studies were performed using 2 nM [^{3}H]Ro5-4864, a concentration where approximately 85% of the specifically bound radioligand was associated with the higher affinity sites expressed after transfection. The rank order of potencies of PK 11195, Ro5-4864, diazepam, clonazepam, and protoporphyrin IX to compete against specific [^{3}H]Ro5-4864 binding (Fig. 6) was consistent with that reported for PBR (17). In parallel experiments Ro5-4864 competed against [^{3}H]PK 11195 binding (2 nM) to membranes of transfected cells with an IC_{50} of about 120 nM (data not shown). This finding is in correspondence with the previous Scatchard analysis (Fig. 5) where it was shown that transfected cells contain two classes of binding sites for PK 11195 displaying different affinities for Ro5-4864. Therefore, PK 11195 and Ro5-4864 reciprocate in competing against the binding of each other to the expressed sites as is characteristic of PBR.

DISCUSSION

The experiments described in this report elaborate on how the photoaffinity probe PK 14105 was used to identify and purify a specific protein associated with PBR. This protein, which is called PKBS, was purified to apparent homogeneity from rat adrenal mitochondrial membranes. Partial amino acid sequencing of peptide fragments derived from PKBS enabled us to clone a cDNA encoding this protein from a rat adrenal library.

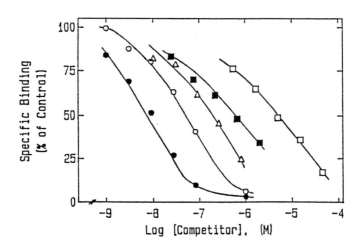

FIGURE 6

Inhibition of [3H]Ro5-4864 binding in transfected cells by different ligands. Nonradioactive PK 11195 (●), Ro5-4864 (O), diazepam (Δ), clonazepam (□), and protoporphyrin IX (■) were tested for inhibition of specific [3H]Ro5-4864 binding (2 nM) to homogenates of transfected 293 cells. Data are presented as the mean of triplicate assays.

The amino acid sequence deduced for PKBS from the cDNA predicts a molecular weight for the protein which is close to the value observed for the protein identified in several tissues (2). The PKBS sequence contains five potential transmembrane-spanning regions with only slight (and possibly insignificant) similarity with subunits comprising the $GABA_A$/benzodiazepine receptor complex. Considerable sequence similarities with proteins in several databases were not found, therefore, at present the PKBS sequence provides no simple clues concerning the biochemical function of PBR.

PKBS is specifically photolabeled by PK 14105 suggesting an intimate relationship between this protein and the binding site for isoquinoline carboxamides. More definitive proof that PKBS comprises the binding domains for PBR ligands is provided by transfection of the human 293 cell line with the pSV-(rat)PKBS expression vector. This results in the elevated expression of about 1 pmol/mg of protein in binding sites for PK 11195 and Ro5-4864 with affinities which are distinctly higher than those observed in control 293 cells. Furthermore, these expressed binding sites exhibit the same rank order of potency for different compounds which interact with PBR. These criteria demonstrate that the sites expressed following transfection with pSV-PKBS exhibit the fundamental properties of PBR.

Previously two other groups had reported that proteins of 30-35 kDa are labeled by two different benzodiazepine affinity-probes believed to modify PBR (25,31). The findings of the work presented here raise the question whether these other protein(s) constitute the benzodiazepine binding domain of PBR. The possibility that PKBS is required to reveal cryptic binding sites on another protein(s) cannot be discounted at this point. The present data do not favor this scheme because, in addition to the photolabeling of PKBS by PK 14105, the transfection studies provide additional evidence supporting the proposal that PKBS contains binding sites for isoquinoline carboxamides and benzodiazepines. First, stoichiometric increases in B_{max} for PK 11195 and Ro5-4864 are observed. Secondly, the affinity of the expressed sites for Ro5-4864 is characteristic of rat PBR rather than that of the human species (4) from which 293 cells were derived. Therefore, the benzodiazepine binding site expressed appears to correspond to the species from which the PKBS cDNA was cloned.

Prior to this work pharmacological probes were the only tools available for studying PBR. The cloning of the PKBS cDNA provides us with a significantly new probe and will now permit new approaches to investigate the cellular functions of PBR.

REFERENCES

1. Anholt, R.R.H., Pedersen, P.L., De Souza, E.B., and Snyder, S.H. (1986): *J. Biol. Chem.*, **261**:576-583.

2. Antkiewicz-Michaluk, L., Guidotti, A., and Krueger, K.E. (1988): *Mol. Pharmacol.*, **34**:272-278.

3. Antkiewicz-Michaluk, L., Mukhin, A.G., Guidotti, A., and Krueger, K.E. (1988): *J. Biol. Chem.*, **263**: 17317-17321.

4. Awad, M. and Gavish, M. (1987): *J. Neurochem.*, **49**: 1407-1414.

5. Benavides, J., Begassat, F., Phan, T., Tur, C., Uzan, A., Renault, C., Dubroeucq, M.C., Gueremy, C., and Le Fur, G. (1984): *Life Sci.*, **35**:1249-1256.

6. Braestrup, C., and Squires, R.F. (1977): *Proc. Natl. Acad. Sci. U.S.A.*, **74**:3805-3809.

7. Costa, E., and Guidotti, A. (1979): *Ann. Rev. Pharmacol. Toxicol.*, **19**:531-545.

8. Costa, E., Guidotti, A., Mao, C.C., and Suria, A. (1975): *Life Sci.*, **17**:167-186.

9. Costa, R.H., Lai, E., and Darnell, J.E. (1986): *Mol. Cell. Biol.*, **6**:4697-4708.

10. Doble, A., Benavides, J., Ferris, O., Bertrand, P., Menager, J., Vaucher, N., Burgevin, M.C., Uzan, A., Gueremy, C. and Le Fur, G. (1985): *Eur J. Pharmacol.*, **119**:153-167.

11. Doble, A., Ferris, O., Burgevin, M.C., Menager, J., Uzan, A., Dubroeucq, M.C., Renault, C., Gueremy, C., and Le Fur, G. (1987): *Mol. Pharmacol.*, **31**:42-49.

12. Dubroeucq, M.C., Benavides, J., Doble, A., Guilloux, F., Allam, D., Vaucher, N., Bertrand, P., Gueremy, C., Renault, C., Uzan, A., and Le Fur, G. (1986): *Eur. J. Pharmacol.*, **128**:269-272.

13. Eisenberg, D., Schwarz, E., Komaromy, M., and Wall, R. (1984): *J. Mol. Biol.*, **179**:125-142.

14. Gallager, D.W., Mallorga, P., Oertel, W., Henneberry, R., and Tallman, J.F. (1981): *J. Neurosci.*, **1**:218-225.

15. Grayson, D.R., Costa, R.H., Xanthopoulos, K.G., and Darnell, J.E. (1988): *Mol. Cell. Biol.*, **8**:1055-1066.

16. Hirsch, J.D., Beyer, C.F., Malkowitz, L., Beer, B., and Blume, A.L. (1989): *Mol. Pharmacol.* **35**:157-163.

17. Hirsch, J.D., Beyer, C.F., Malkowitz, L., Loullis, C.C., and Blume, A.L. (1989): *Mol. Pharmacol.*, **35**:164-172.

18. Klein, P., Kanethsa, M., and Delisi, C. (1985): *Biochem. Biophys. Acta,* **815**:468-476.

19. Kyte, J. and Doolittle, R.F. (1982): *J. Mol. Biol.*, **157**:105-132.

20. Laemlli, U.K. (1970): *Nature,* **227**:680-685.

21. Langer, S.Z. and Arbilla, S. (1988): *Pharmacol. Biochem. Behav.*, **29**:763-766.

22. Le Fur, G., Perrier, M.L., Vaucher, N., Imbault, F., Flamier, A., Uzan, A., Renault, C., Dubroeucq, M.C., and Gueremy, C. (1983): *Life Sci.*, **32**:1839-1847.

23. Lukeman, D.S. and Fanestil, D.D. (1987): *J. Pharmacol. Exp. Ther.*, **241**:950-955.

24. Marangos, P.J., Patel, J., Boulenger, J.P., and Clark-Rosenberg, R. (1982): *Mol. Pharmacol.*, **22**:26-32.

25. McCabe, R.T., Schoenheimer, J.A., Skolnick, P., Hauck-Newman, A., Rice, K.C., Reig, J.-A., and Klein, D.C. (1989): *FEBS Letters*, **244**:263-267.

26. Olson M., Ciliax, B.J., Mancini, W.R., and Young, A.B. (1988): *Eur. J. Pharmacol.*, **152**:47-53.

27. Paul, S.M., Kempner, E.S., and Skolnick, P. (1981): *Eur. J. Pharmacol.*, **76**:465-466.

28. Pritchett, D.B., Sontheimer, H., Shivers, B.D., Ymer, S., Kettenmann, H., Schofield, P.R., and Seeburg, P.H. (1989): *Nature*, **338**:582-585.

29. Schofield, P.R., Darlison, M.G., Fujita, N., Burt, D.R., Stephenson, F.A., Rodriguez, H., Rhee, L.M., Ramachandran, J., Reale, V., Glencorse, T., Seeburg, P.H., and Barnard, E.A. (1987): *Nature*, **328**: 221-227.

30. Skowronski, R., Beaumont, K., and Fanestil, D.D. (1987): *Eur. J. Pharmacol.*, **143**:305-314.

31. Snyder, S.H., Verma, A., and Trifiletti, R.R. (1987): *FASEB* J., **1**:282-288.

32. Valtier, D., Malgouris, C., Gilbert, J.-C., Guicheney, P., Uzan, A., Gueremy, C., Le Fur, G., Saraux, H., and Meyer, P. (1987): *Neuropharmacology*, **26**:549-554.

33. Verma, A. and Snyder, S.H. (1988): *Mol. Pharmacol.*, **34**:800-805.

34. Wang, J.K., Taniguchi, T., and Spector, S. (1984): *Mol. Pharmacol.*, **25**:349-351

GABA and Benzodiazepine Receptor Subtypes,
edited by Giovanni Biggio and Erminio Costa.
Raven Press, New York © 1990.

ELUCIDATING GABA$_A$ RECEPTOR HETEROGENEITY: AN INTEGRATED MOLECULAR APPROACH

Peter H. Seeburg

Laboratory of Molecular Neuroendocrinology, ZMBH, University of Heidelberg, Im Neuenheimer Feld 282, 6900 Heidelberg, FRG

Introduction

Many small molecule neurotransmitters interact with members of two very different families of neuroreceptors, those containing intrinsic ion channels whose activity is gated by the neurotransmitter (ionotropic) and those activating G proteins to access the metabolic machinery of target cells (metabotropic). For γ-aminobutyric acid (GABA), the major inhibitory neurotransmitter in the vertebrate nervous system, the ion channel is designated as the GABA$_A$ receptor (for review, see ref. 13) and the G protein-coupled receptor, as the GABA$_B$ receptor. In keeping with the molecular design of other ligand-gated ion channels (for review, see ref. 26), the GABA$_A$ receptor consists of subunits which assemble to form the functional receptor/ion channel. The GABA$_A$ receptor/channel conducts chloride ions and can be activity-modulated by a variety of clinically relevant psychoactive compounds of which benzodiazepines and barbiturates are among the best-known examples (13).

A purification scheme based on high affinity benzodiazepine binding sites located on the GABA$_A$ receptor complex permitted an initial biochemical characterization of this receptor (5, 18, 24). Specifically, several subunits can be resolved by gel electrophoresis of the purified complex and a subset of these can be visualized (6, 23) by the use of photoreactive benzodiazepine derivatives (12). Partial amino acid sequences of two subunits determined by micro-sequencing permitted us to describe a large part of the natural heterogeneity of GABA$_A$ receptors by molecular cloning techniques (1, 9, 14, 17, 19, 22, 29, 30). The following outlines our approach to study the molecular and functional complexity of GABA$_A$ receptors.

GABA~A~ receptor subunits

All GABA$_A$ receptor subunits are homologous and belong to the superfamily of subunits for ligand-gated ion channels which includes the subunits of the nicotinic acetylcholine receptor, the glycine receptor, and, presumably, the glutamate and serotonin 5HT-3 receptors (26). These subunits are 450-550 residue polypeptides with four transmembrane segments (TMI to TMIV), three in the middle of the molecule and one at the C-terminus. Approximately the N-terminal half of each subunit is predicted to be extracellularly located. It contains N-linked glycosylation sites and a 15 residue ß-structural disulfide-bonded loop of unknown function. The region between TMIII and TMIV is intracellularly located and displays the highest sequence divergence, even between closely related subunits.

We and others have isolated cloned cDNAs for 12 different GABA$_A$ receptor subunits from human, rat and bovine species (1, 8-11. 14, 17, 19, 20, 22, 29, 30). These subunits can be arranged in distinct classes according to sequence and function with one to several variants in each class (22). The α subunit class so far comprises six variants, there are three different ß subunits, two γ subunits and only one δ subunit. While we expect that more α subunit variants may be found we are reasonably certain that only two γ subunits and one δ subunit exist. The degree of sequence similarity between members of different subunit classes is 30-40% and variants within a given class share 70-80% sequence indentity. The complexity of GABA$_A$ receptor subunits is suggestive of functional heterogeneity. In particular, the unexpectedly large number of α subunit variants indicates the existence of different populations of GABA$_A$ receptors in which the α subunit variants substitute for each other. Within the framework of this model, we should expect a differential temporal and spatial distribution of α subunits in the CNS of developing and mature animals (see below).

Functional expression

The observed complexity of GABA$_A$ receptor subunits can be conveniently studied by the use of an efficient expression system for assessing the functionality of these subunits. We adapted a transient expression system in cultured mammalian cells, originally developed by C. Gorman (7), to express single subunits and their combinations (16, 17). The receptors formed by the assembly of subunits were analyzed by both pharmacology and electrophysiology and the results permitted a direct comparison to previously described properties of central GABA$_A$ receptors.

Molecular pharmacology and electrophysiology

High-affinity binding sites for several classes of compounds exist on natural $GABA_A$ receptors. We assayed for the presence of such binding sites on various recombinant receptors. The minimal requirement for high-affinity [^{3}H]muscimol binding was met by the coexpression of two different subunits, α and β, or, α and γ_2 subunits (17). Receptors formed by the assembly of single subunits did not contain measurable [^{3}H]muscimol binding sites, although such receptors showed GABA-evoked chloride currents.

An important characteristic of natural $GABA_A$ receptors is the presence of high-affinity benzodiazepine binding sites (13). These sites can be generated <u>in vitro</u> by the coexpression of three subunits (17). The most consistent results are obtained upon coexpression of any of several α variants with a β subunit and γ subunit. Combinations of two subunits have not been seen to produce receptors displaying measurable benzodiazepine binding. However, as detailed below, the presence of high-affinity benzodiazepine binding sites does not always correlate with the benzodiazepine-mediated stimulation of GABA-evoked chloride currents.

$GABA_A$ receptor-associated benzodiazepine binding sites have been grouped into two pharmacological types, BZI- and BZII-sites (4, 13). The distinction between these sites is possible by their differential affinities of certain compounds e.g., CL 218872 and 2-oxo-quazepam. These bind with a higher affinity to BZI sites. Our recombinant expression studies showed that the differential affinities can be mimicked by the substitution of certain α subunit variants. Thus, the α_1 subunit in combination with a β variant and the γ_2 subunit creates BZI site pharmacology whereas the α_2, α_3 or α_5 variant generates BZII sites when coexpressed with these same β and γ subunits (14, 15, 17). These results clearly show that, at a minimum, BZII sites are heterogeneous, consisting of a mixture of receptor populations (14, 15). The alignment of the α subunit variants shows distinct sequence differences in regions such as the extracellular domain where benzodiazepines may bind. We are currently investigating the effects of amino acid substitutions in this region of the molecule on benzodiazepine affinities.

Upon transfection, approximately one-half of the cultured cells transiently express $GABA_A$ receptors. These cells can be analysed by whole-cell patch clamp techniques regarding the channel properties and the pharmacology of recombinant $GABA_A$ receptors. Results from these studies can be correlated with the electrophysiological properties of natural GABA_A receptors. The following summarizes the salient features of recombinant GABA-gated channels.

GABA evokes chloride channels in cultured cells expressing single subunits (17, 22). This is true for member of all subunit classes and, in fact, constitutes an important functional criterion to include novel subunits to the growing family of GABA_A receptor subunits (22). These "homomeric" channels exhibit a distinct rudimentary GABA-ergic pharmacology. Thus, GABA-evoked channel activity is reversibly repressed in the presence of bicuculline and picrotoxin and can be potentiated by the barbiturate, pentobarbital. However, neither homomeric receptors, nor receptors assembled from only α and β subunits show consistent responses to benzodiazepines or to negative modulaters e.g., DMCM. Only the benzodiazepine antagonist, Ro15-1788, enhances GABA-mediated currents at elevated concentrations.

In contrast, recombinant receptors containing the γ_2 subunit show a pronounced reactivity towards benzodiazepines e.g., flunitrazepam and diazepam. Also, in such receptors, DMCM at low concentrations diminishes GABA-evoked currents, as seen in mammalian GABA_A receptors (16).

Natural GABA_A receptors display a variety of conductance states (2, 3, 25). By contrast, recombinant receptors assembled from two or three subunits show a limited range of conductance state and one main state. This state differs for receptors formed by α and β subunits (20 pS) relative to receptors formed by α and γ subunits (30 pS) (ref. 27). A combination of β and γ subunits usually results in small GABA-evoked currents and hence, this combination has not been studied further. The fact that recombinant receptors display a limited range of conductance states suggests that "natural" receptors may consist of receptor populations, with each population characterized by one defined conductance state.

Localization of subunits

Two complementary methods are currently in use to analyse the spatial and temporal expression pattern of GABA_A receptor subunits in the CNS, immunocytochemistry and in situ hybridization. Since, at present, subunit specific antibodies need constructing, we and others have made use of the available nucleotide sequence information to develop subunit specific tools for in situ hybridization (17, 21, 22, 28). This technique, although lacking spatial resolution to determine differential cellular localization of receptor populations, nevertheless is extremely useful to determine which of the genes for the subunits are expressed in different neural cell populations. Importantly, the mRNAs encoding the three α subunit variants α_1, α_2 and α_3 are expressed differentially in brain regions, consistent with the notion that these subunits define BZI and BZII receptors. Furthermore, mRNAs encoding two novel subunits, γ_2 and δ were seen to be widely expressed and present often in different but overlapping neuronal cell populations, suggesting that these subunits define distinct receptor subtypes (22). Of these, the receptors containing the γ_2 subunit may be present in GABA_A receptors with high affinity benzodiazepine binding sites. Further studies will show the developmental regulation of GABA_A receptor subunits and provide evidence for the expression of several receptor subtypes by the same neurons, e.g. the Purkinje cells on the spinal cord motor neurons.

Outlook

The experiments described here are directed to evaluate the structural and functional heterogeneity of central GABA_A/benzodiazepine receptors. While molecular cloning approaches result in the characterization of receptor subunits and their variants, expression studies coupled with pharmacological and electrophysiological analyses are needed to study the full functional spectrum of receptors formed by subunit combinations.

However, due to the plasticity of subunit assembly which may permit the formation of receptors from subunits which are not co-expressed in vivo, these studies need complementary evaluations concerning the natural expression patterns of receptor subunits. In addition, functional studies of these receptors in in vivo situations as provided by recently-developed slice-technique are of crucial importance. Combined, all these efforts are directed to describe the set of naturally occurring GABA_A receptors, their composition and their function. Results will permit the construction of a set of cell lines expressing the complete panel of GABA_A receptor subtypes. This panel should prove invaluable for the design and development of subtype specific ligands with minimal cross-reactivity for the clinical treatment of e.g. epilepsy, anxiety and memory deficits.

Acknowledgements

The author acknowledges the excellent secretarial help provided by Jutta Rami. The work of the laboratory summarized in this chapter was funded by grants of the Deutsche Forschungsgemeinschaft and the Bundesministerium für Forschung und Technologie.

References

1. Barnard, E.A., Darlison, M.G., and Seeburg, P.H. (1987): *TINS* 10: 502-509.
2. Bormann, J. and Clapham, D.E. (1985): *Proc. Natl. Acad. Sci. U.S.A.* 82: 2168-2172.
3. Bormann, J., Hamill, O.P., and Sakmann, B. (1987): *J. Physiol.* 385: 243-286.
4. Braestrup, C. and Squires, R.F. (1977) *Proc. Natl. Acad. Sci. U.S.A.,* 74: 3805-3809.
5. Casalotti, S.O., Stephenson, F.A., and Barnard, E.A. (1986): *J. Biol. Chem.* 261: 15013-15016.
6. Fuchs, K., Möhler, H., and Sieghart, W. (1988): *Neuroscience Lett.* 90: 314-319.
7. Gorman, C.M., Gier, D., McGray, G., and Huang, M. (1989): *Virology* 171: 377-385.
8. Khrestchatisky, M., MacLennan, A.J., Chiang, M.-Y., Xu, W., Jackson, M.B., Brecha, N., Stermini, C., Olsen, R.W., and Tobin, A.J. (1989): *Neuron* 3: 745-753.
9. Levitan, E.S., Schofield, P.R., Burt, D.R., Rhee, L.M., Wisden, W., Koehler, M., Rodriguez, H., Stephenson, F.A., Darlison, M.G., Barnard, E.A., and Seeburg, P.H. (1988): *Nature* 335: 76-79.
10. Lolait, S.J., O'Caroll, A.M., Kusano, K., Muller, J.M., Brownstein, M.J., and Mahan, L.C. (1989): *FEBS Lett.* 246: 145-148.
11. Malherbe, P., Sigel, E., Baur, R., Persohn, E., Richards, J.G. and Möhler, H. (1990): *FEBS Lett.* 280: 261-265.
12. Möhler, H. and Okada, T (1977): *Science* 198: 849-851.
13. Olsen, R.W. and Venter, J.C. (1986): *Benzodiazepine/GABA receptors and Chloride Channels: Structural and Functional Properties.* Liss, New York.
14. Pritchett, D.B. and Seeburg, P.H. (1990): *J. Neurochem.* in press.
15. Pritchett, D.B., Lüddens, H., and Seeburg, P.H. (1989): *Science* 245: 1389-1392.
16. Pritchett, D.B., Sontheimer, H., Gorman, C.M., Kettenmann, H., Seeburg, and Schofield, P.R. (1988): *Science* 242: 1306-1309.
17. Pritchett, D.B., Sontheimer, H., Shivers, B.D., Ymer, S., Kettenmann, H., Schofield, P.R., and Seeburg, P.H. (1989): *Nature* 338: 582-585.
18. Schoch, P., Häring, P., Takacs, B., Stähli, C., and Möhler, H. (1984): *J. Recept. Res.* 4: 198-200.
19. Schofield, P.R., Darlison, M.G., Fujita, N., Rodriguez, H.,Burt, D.R., Stephenson, F.A., Rhee, L.M., Ramachandran, J., Glencorse, T.A., Reale, V., Seeburg, P.H., and Barnard, E.A. (1987): *Nature* 328: 221-227.
20. Schofield, P.R., Pritchett, D.B., Sontheimer, H., Kettenmann, H., and Seeburg, P.H. (1989): *FEBS Lett.* 244: 361-364.

21. Séquier, J.M., Richards, J.G.,. Malherbe, P., Price, G.W., Mathews, and Möhler, H. (1988): *Proc. Natl. Acad. Sci. U.S.A.* 85: 7815-7819.
22. Shivers, B.D., Killisch, I., Sprengel, R., Sontheimer, H., Köhler, M., Schofield, P.R., and Seeburg, P.H. (1989): *Neuron* 3: 327-337.
23. Sieghart, W. and Karobath, M. (1980): *Nature* 286: 285-287.
24. Sigel, E., Stephenson, F.A., Mamalaki, C., and Barnard, E.A. (1983): *J. Biol. Chem.* 258: 6965-6971.
25. Smith, S.M., Zoree, R., and McBurney, R.N. (1989): *J. Membrane Biol.* 180: 45-52.
26. Unwin, N. (1989): *Neuron*: 3: 665-676.
27. Verdoorn, T.A., Draguhn, A., Ymer, S., Seeburg, P.H., and Sakmann, B. (1990): *Neuron*, in press.
28. Wisden, W., Morris, B.J., Darlison, M.G., Hunt, S.P., and Barnard, E.A. (1987): *Molecular Brain Res.* 5: 505-310.
29. Ymer, S., Draguhn, A., Köhler, M., Schofield, P.R., and Seeburg, P.H. (1989): *FEBS Lett.* 258: 119-122.
30. Ymer, S., Schofield, P.R., Draguhn, A., Werner, P., Köhler, M., and Seeburg, P.H. (1989): *EMBO J.* 8: 1665-1670.

GABA and Benzodiazepine Receptor Subtypes,
edited by Giovanni Biggio and Erminio Costa.
Raven Press, New York © 1990.

GABA$_A$-RECEPTOR SUBUNITS: FUNCTIONAL EXPRESSION AND GENE LOCALISATION

H. Mohler[+], P. Malherbe, A. Draguhn[*], E. Sigel[x], J.M. Sequier,
E. Persohn and J.G. Richards

Pharmaceutical Research Department, F. Hoffmann-La Roche Ltd,
Basel, Switzerland
[*]Max-Planck-Institut für Medizinische Forschung, Heidelberg,FRG
[x]Institute of Pharmacology, University of Bern, Switzerland
[+]Present address: Institute of Pharmacology, University of Zürich,
Switzerland

The GABA$_A$-receptor is a heterooligomeric synaptic protein complex which constitutes a gated chloride channel. Through its allosteric modulation by drugs its serves as a molecular control element for the regulation of anxiety, vigilance, muscle tension and epileptiform activity (3, 4). Two protein components, the α- and ß-subunit, were identified as main constituents of the affinity-purified receptor (13, 16, 17, 20). However, it is unclear whether these two proteins constitute a fully functional GABA$_A$-receptor and how they can account for receptor heterogeneity. Molecular cloning of subunit cDNAs and their functional expression might provide new insights into the structure and possible function of multiple GABA$_A$-receptors in the brain. This experimental approach led to the recognition of three classes of subunits (α, ß, γ) which are characterized by a 30-35 % sequence identity (7, 10, 11, 14). Within each class rather homologous variants exist which show a 70-75 % sequence identity (6). Our group has isolated cDNAs coding for six α-subunits, two ß-subunits and one γ-subunit in rat brain. The subunit heterogeneity observed arises from different genes encoding various polypeptides and variants thereof and are not generated by alternative splicing.

23

In the following the functional properties of recombinant receptors will be described which were expressed from various subunit cDNAs in Xenopus oocytes. In addition, the sites of subunit gene expression in situ are outlined with the aim to identify those subunit combinations which are co-expressed in vivo in specified neuronal populations. The heterogeneity of GABA_A-receptors in the brain may contribute to synaptic plasticity, differential responsiveness of neurons to GABA and to variations in drug profiles.

RECOMBINANT RECEPTORS EXPRESSED FROM α_1- AND β_1-SUBUNIT cDNAS OF RAT BRAIN

Molecular cloning of the α_1- and β_1-subunit cDNAs provided information on the topology of the GABA_A-receptor polypeptides in the membrane (Fig. 1, ref. 8, 14).

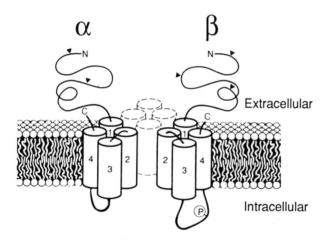

Fig. 1 Model of the topology of the GABA_A-receptor α- and ß-subunits. Putative membrane-spanning helices are depicted as cylinders. Potential sites for N-glycosylation are indicated by triangles. A consensus site for serine phosphorylation by protein-kinase A, which is present only in the β-subunit, is indicated by an encircled P.

In order to determine the functional properties of the recombinant receptors generated from the rat brain α_1- and β_1-subunits, the corresponding subunit RNAs were expressed in Xenopus oocytes and currents were recorded under voltage clamp at -70 mV (7). About 90 % of the RNA-injected oocytes showed dose-dependent inward currents in response to the application of GABA (Fig. 2). The current was due to gated chloride channels since its reversal potential was −20.5 mV, close to the chloride equilibrium potential under the recording conditions. Furthermore, the GABA-induced current response was inhibited in the presence of the GABA-antagonist bicuculline. Since GABA-induced current responses were previously observed even with homomeric channels expressed from either α_1- or β_1-subunits (10), binding sites for GABA appear to be located on both the α- and β-subunits.

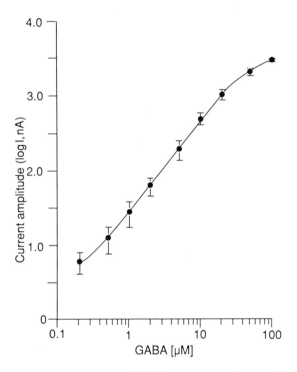

Fig. 2 Relationship between GABA concentration (µM, log scale) and current amplitude (nA, log scale). Data are means ± SD from three different oocytes co-injected with α_1- and β_1-subunit RNAs.

POTENTIATION AND ACTIVATION BY PENTOBARBITAL

Potentiation by barbiturates is a key feature of the native GABA$_A$-receptor. It was retained in the recombinant receptor expressed from rat brain α_1 + β_1-subunits (Fig. 3). For instance, at

2 μM GABA the current amplitude was increased in the presence of 25 μM pentobarbital by 350 ± 200 % (n=6). Pentobarbital alone (25 μM) had little direct effect (< 20nA). These results are consistent with earlier findings on recombinant receptors formed by the coexpression of α_1- and β_1-subunits of bovine and human brain (10, 14).

High concentrations of pentobarbital (100 μM) elicited inward currents at the recombinant α_1 + β_1-receptor even in the absence of GABA and thus directly activate the recombinant receptor. This property is shared with the native receptor (3) and the recombinant receptor expressed from bovine (5, 14) but not human (10) α_1- and β_1-subunits.

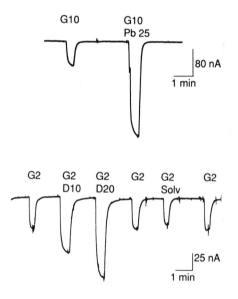

Fig. 3 Potentiation of the GABA-induced membrane current by various drugs in oocytes co-injected with rat α_1- and β_1-subunit RNAs. Downward deflections represent inward currents measured under voltage clamp at -70 mV. GABA (G) was applied alone at 2 or 10 μM (G 2, G 10) or in combination with (top) pentobarbital 25 μM (Pb 25) or (below) diazepam 10 and 20 μM (D, 10,20). The solvent of diazepam (Solv) was without effect.

ATYPICAL MODULATION BY LIGANDS OF THE BENZODIAZEPINE RECEPTOR

The benzodiazepine receptor site is unique in that it mediates two opposite pharmacological effects, facilitation as well as reduction of GABA$_A$-receptor function. This property is not only observed at native GABA$_A$-receptors (3, 4) but also in oocytes injected with whole brain RNA (18). It was therefore tested whether this modulatory ability was retained in GABA$_A$-receptors which were expressed in oocytes from α_1- and β_1-subunit cDNAs of rat brain. The GABA-induced current response of the recombinant receptor was potentiated in a dose-dependent manner in the presence of various tranquillizing benzodiazepines (diazepam, flunitrazepam and midazolam) in 20 out of 31 oocytes tested (7 independent injections) (7). For instance, at 2 μM GABA the current was potentiated in the presence of 10 and 20 μM diazepam by 45 $\pm$ 21 % (n=8), and 93 $\pm$ 46 % (n=5) respectively (Fig. 3). The benzodiazepine antagonist flumazenil (10 μM) despite its very weak agonistic intrinsic activity in vivo (2), likewise potentiated the GABA-response. At 2 and 10 μM GABA the current amplitude was increased by 75 %. Most surprisingly, the β-carboline DMCM, which acts as an inverse agonist of the benzodiazepine receptor in neuronal tissue (3, 4) as well as in oocytes injected with whole brain RNA (18), potentiated the GABA-response of the recombinant receptor. At 2 μM GABA the response was potentiated in the presence of DMCM (10 μM) by 67 $\pm$ 22 % (n=3), at 10 mM GABA by 43 $\pm$ 40 % (n =3). Thus, it can be concluded that GABA$_A$-receptors expressed in oocytes from α_1 + β_1-subunits of rat brain contain benzodiazepine binding sites as shown by the modulation of their GABA response by diazepam, flumazenil and DMCM. The mechanism of signal transduction is, however, not fully operational, since both the antagonist flumazenil as well as DMCM potentiated the GABA-response.

The results obtained with receptors expressed from α_1 + β_1-subunits of rat brain are in striking contrast to those obtained with the corresponding bovine and human α_1- and β_1-subunits (5, 6, 10) where neither a reproducible potentiation of the GABA-response with agonists nor a response to inverse agonists was found. This functional discrepancy between the receptors expressed from α_1- and β_1-subunits of different species cannot be readily explained at present. The small differences in primary sequences of the cloned subunits may be sufficient to affect protein processing and assembly in the oocytes leading to functionally divergent receptors. Alternatively, heterogeneity among oocytes may have to be considered. While responses to GABA can be recorded in >95% of RNA-injected oocytes diazepam potentiation of the GABA-reponse was only seen in 60 % of the cells responding to GABA. Thus, not all oocytes seem to fulfill the requirements needed for the processing and assembly of subunits into a benzodiazepine-sensitive receptor. Indeed, differences in the expression repertoire among different batches and sources of oocytes are known (1).

EVIDENCE FOR COOPERATIVITY OF GABA

Injection of total poly(A)+RNA of brain into Xenopus oocytes leads to the expression of GABA$_A$-receptors with maximal slopes of the GABA dose-response curves of 1.4 (9, 18) or 1.7 (19) which is close to the value of the native receptor in spinal cord neurons (12). When the cDNAs coding for the α_1- and β_1-subunits of rat brain were expressed in Xenopus oocytes, evidence for cooperativity could be found (7). The maximal slopes of the double logarithmic plots of the GABA dose-response data yielded a mean slope of 1.2 ± 0.1 (n=3) between 2 and 20 μM GABA (Fig. 2). Since desensitization became apparent at GABA concentrations higher than 10 μM true maximal current amplitudes were probably not reached at higher GABA concentrations and the slopes of the dose-response data might be underestimated. Non-desensitizing conditions e.g. fast application of GABA, may have to be established in order to quantify GABA-cooperativity.

It is presently unexplained why recombinant receptor expressed from bovine and human α_1- and β_1-subunits showed no evidence for GABA-cooperativity (5, 10, 14). It is particularly surprising that receptors expressed from α_1-, β_1- and γ_2-subunit, which display functional benzodiazepine receptor sites (see below), yielded no evidence for GABA cooperativity (11). Thus, conflicting data exist at present on the structural requirements for the cooperativity of GABA in activating the chloride channel.

RECOMBINANT RECEPTORS WITH FUNCTIONAL BENZODIAZEPINE RECEPTOR SITES

Recombinant GABA$_A$-receptors which display functional benzodiazepine receptor sites were recently generated by the co-expression of human α_1-, β_1- and γ_2-subunit cDNAs in cultured mammalian cells (11). GABA-induced responses (5-10 μM) were enhanced about two fold by the agonists diazepam and flunitrazepam (2 μM) and reduced by 50 % in the presence of the inverse agonist DMCM (1 μM). This result was qualitatively confirmed by our group by expression in Xenopus oocytes of RNA coding for the α_1-, β_1- and γ_2-subunits of rat brain. However, the extent of the drug-induced modulation of the GABA response was much less pronounced than in the experiments described above. The response to GABA (2.5 μM) was enhanced in the presence of diazepam (1 μM) by only 17 ± 7 % (n=11) and reduced by DMCM (0.3 μM) by only 6 ± 4 % (n=6) although drug concentrations were used which yielded maximum modulatory effects at oocytes injected with whole brain chick RNA (18). Whether these discrepancies in the extent of the drug-responses at the recombinant receptors of human and rat brain are due to the species difference of the subunit cDNAs or due to differences in the expression systems remains to be clarified. Nevertheless, it is noteworthy that the $\alpha_1 + \beta_1 + \gamma_2$-receptors respond to allosteric modulation by ligands of the benzodiazepine receptor at somewhat lower concentrations than the $\alpha_1 + \beta_1$-receptors.

The full structural requirements for a functional GABA$_A$-receptor are still elusive. Although co-expression of the α_1-, β_1- and γ_2-subunits yields recombinant receptors which respond to positive and negative allosteric modulation at the benzodiazepine receptor, no evidence for cooperativity in gating the channel was found (11). Furthermore, it is conceivable that subunits other than γ_2 may also convey sensitivity to benzodiazepine receptor ligands. Despite prominent expression of γ_2-mRNA in major neuronal population in the brain, the γ_2-subunit does not appear to be co-expressed in all neurons expressing α_1- and β_1-subunits (see below). Thus, subunit combinations other than α_1, β_1, γ_2 would be expected to generate GABA$_A$-receptors with functional benzodiazepine receptor sites.

VARIANTS OF THE α-SUBUNIT CONVEY DIFFERENTIAL SENSITIVITY TO GABA

The heterogeneity of GABA$_A$-receptor subunits is particularly apparent for the α-subunit of which six variant cDNAs have been isolated. In order to test whether the multiplicity of α-subunits is of possible functional relevance, various α-subunit cDNAs were co-expressed with the β_1-subunit in Xenopus oocytes. Some of the recombinant receptors displayed striking differences in their sensitivity to GABA. For instance, the receptor expressed from α_5 +

ß_1-subunits showed a half-maximal response at about 10^{-6}M GABA, while the α_1 + ß_1-combination showed an approximately 10-fold lower sensitivity to GABA. These results extend earlier observations with three α-subunit variants of bovine brain (α_1, α_2, α_3), which were likewise distinguished by their apparent sensitivity to GABA when expressed with the ß_1-subunit (6). Since the genes for at least some α-subunit variants are expressed independently in different neuronal populations (see below) they may convey a differential GABA-responsiveness to these neurons in vivo.

GENES OF THE α_1-, ß_1- AND γ_2-SUBUNITS ARE CO-EXPRESSED IN SOME BRAIN AREAS

Mapping the pattern of subunit gene expression by in situ hybridization histochemistry is expected to identify the types of subunit combinations which may give rise to GABA_A-receptor heterogeneity in defined neuronal populations. Furthermore, studies on subunit gene expression may provide new insights into possible variations of subunit expression under altered physiological or pathological conditions. Alterations in receptor structure might be part of the functional adaptation of GABAergic synapses.

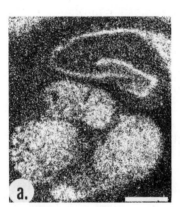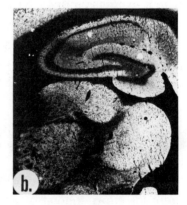

Fig. 4 Site of transcription and translation of the α_1-subunit gene as visualized in parasaggital sections of rat brain. a) In situ hybridization with the ^{35}S-labeled cRNA antisense strand of the α_1-subunit. b) Immunohistochemical staining of the receptor protein by the monoclonal antibody bd-17 (Bar= 1 mm).

Initially, the distribution of α_1- and β_1-subunit mRNA was visualized and compared with the immunohistochemical staining of the receptor protein in rat brain sections (15). The correspondence between receptor density and the hybridzation intensity was particularly striking with the α_1-subunit probe - e.g. in the main and accessory olfactory bulb, cerebral cortex, ventral pallidum, globus pallidus, hippocampal formation (Fig. 4), thalamus, substantia nigra, inferior colliculus, and cerebellum. Since the receptor is thought to comprise both α- and ß-subunits, the hybridization pattern of the α_1-subunit probe was compared with that of the β_1-subunit probe. Strong hybridization signals with both the α_1- and β_1-subunit probes were found in several brain areas known to contain high densities of GABA~A~ receptors   e.g. cerebral cortex and hippocampal formation (Fig. 5).

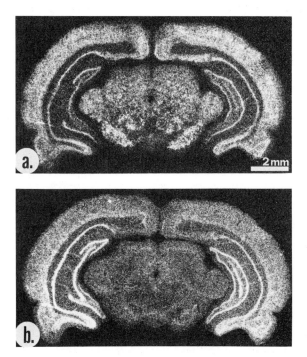

Fig. 5 Expression of the α_1- and the β_1-subunit gene visualized by in situ hybridization histochemistry in frontal sections of rat brain. Comparison between the hybridization pattern obtained with the ^{35}S-labeled RNA antisense strands of a) the α_1-subunit and b) the β_1-subunit. (Bar= 2 mm)

On the level of single neurons, a strong hybridization signal was found with both the α_1- and the ß$_1$-subunit probe in the somata of hippocampal pyramidal neurons, mitral cells of the olfactory bulb, and granule cells of the dentate gyrus and cerebellum. However, in some brain areas that show a high GABA$_A$ receptor content, the intensity of the hybridization signal differed strikingly between the α_1- and ß$_1$-subunit probes.

The ß-probe signal was much weaker than that of the α-probe in, for example, thalamus, inferior colliculus, and substantia nigra. Conversely, the α-probe signal was much weaker than the ß-probe signal in bed nucleus, for example (15).

Thus, variants of α- and ß-subunits were expected to occur in the respective brain areas. Indeed, when the patterns of gene expression of α-subunit variants were mapped, an uneven distribution became apparent. Whereas α_1-mRNA was ubiquitously distributed throughout rat brain, mRNAs for the variants α2, 3, 5, 6 were co-localized apparently only in pyramidal and granule cells of the hippocampal formation. Moreover, with the exception of α5, all α-subtypes were detected in cerebellar granule cells while only α_1 and α2 were unequivocally present in Purkinje cells. All α-subunit variants were expressed in cerebral cortex, although they were differentially distributed among the laminae. Thus, expression of the α-subunit variants is under independent regulatory control.

The γ_2-subunit appears to convey functional benzodiazepine binding sites to recombinant receptors when co-expressed with the α_1- and ß$_1$-subunit cDNAs (see above). Therefore the pattern of gene expression of the γ_2-subunit was mapped and compared to that of the α_1- and ß$_1$-subunits. Major neuronal populations appear to co-express α_1-, ß$_1$- and (albeit somewhat weaker) γ_2-subunit mRNA as shown by the respective hybridization signals in cerebral cortex, olfactory bulb, hippocampal formation and cerebellar granule cells. These findings suggests that the α_1-, ß$_1$- and γ_2-subunits are likely components of the GABA$_A$-receptors in these brain areas. However, in other brain areas e.g. some, but not all, thalamic nuclei, no γ_2 hybridization signal could be detected. Thus, an extensive, yet unresolved, receptor-heterogeneity appears to exist in brain whose functional exploration may open new views on GABAergic synaptic transmission. It may convey a differential responsiveness of neurons to GABA, contribute to synaptic plasticity and may lead to the development of novel drugs which are selective for receptor-subtypes.

OUTLOOK

1) Receptor structure: The factor(s) and subunit(s) which constitute fully functional GABA$_A$-receptor are still elusive. Their identification will be a major aim of future research.

2) Receptor heterogeneity: The clarification of the functional role of subclasses of GABA$_A$-receptors may provide new insights into the role of GABAergic synaptic transmission in defined neuronal populations.

3) Receptor expression: Plasticity of the GABA$_A$-receptor may arise from differential subunit expression under altered physiological or pathological conditions. The investigation of such phenomena may contribute new views on the role of GABAergic transmission in neuronal adaptation and in CNS diseases.

REFERENCES

1. Dascal, N. (1987): *CRC Critical Reviews in Biochemistry*, 22:317-386.
2. Haefely, W. (1988): *Eur. J. Anaesthesiol.*, Supp. 2:25-36.
3. Haefely, W. (1989): In: *Allosteric Modulation of Amino Acid Receptors: Therapeutic Implications*, edited by E.A. Barnard, and E. Costa. pp. 47-70. Raven Press, New York.
4. Haefely, W., Kyburz, E., Gerecke, M., and Mohler, H. (1985): *Adv. Drug Res.*, 14:165-322.
5. Levitan, E.S., Blair, L.A.C., Dionne, V.E., and Barnard, E.A. (1988): *Neuron*, 1:779-781.
6. Levitan, E.S., Schofield, P.R., Burt, D.R., Rhee, L.M., Wisden, W., Kohler, M., Fujita, N., Rodriguez, H.F., Stephenson, S., Darlison, M.G., Barnard, E.A., and Seeburg, P.H. (1988): *Nature*, 335: 76-79.
7. Malherbe, P., Draguhn, A., Multhaup, G., Beyreuther, K., and Mohler, H. (1989): (submitted).
8. Mohler, H., Malherbe, P., Sequier, J.M., Bannwarth, W., Schoch, P., and Richards, J.G. (1989): In: *Allosteric Modulation of Amino Acid Receptors: Therapeutic Implications*, edited by E.A. Barnard, and E. Costa. pp. 31-46. Raven Press, New York.

9. Parker, I., Gundersen, B., and Miledi, R. (1986): *J. Neurosci.*, 6:2290-2297.
10. Pritchett, D.B., Sontheimer, H., Gorman, C.M., Kettenmann, H., Seeburg, P.H., and Schofield, P.R. (1988): *Science*, 242:1306-1308.
11. Pritchett, D.B., Sontheimer, H., Shivers, B.D., Ymer, S., Kettenmann, H., Schofield, P.R., and Seeburg, P.H. (1989): *Nature*, 338:582-585.
12. Sakmann, B., Hamill, O.P., and Bormann, M. (1983): *J. Neural Transm.*, Suppl. 18:83-95.
13. Schoch, P., Häring, P., Takacs, B., Stähli, C., and Mohler, H. (1984): *J. Recept. Res.*, 4:189-200.
14. Schofield, P.R., Darlison, M.G., Fujita, N., Burt, D.R., Stephenson, F.A., Rodriguez, H., Rhee, L.M., Ramachandran, V.R., Glencorse, R., Seeburg, P.H., and Barnard, E.A. (1987): *Nature*, 328:221-227.
15. Sequier, J.M., Richards, J.G., Malherbe, P., Price, G.W., Matthews, S., and Mohler, H. (1988): *Proc. Natl. Acad. Sci. USA*, 85:7815-7819.
16. Sigel, E., Stephenson, F.A., Mamalaki, C., and Barnard, E.A. (1983): *J. Biol. Chem.*, 258:6965-6971.
17. Sigel, E., and Barnard, E.A. (1984): *J. Biol. Chem.*, 259:7219-7223.
18. Sigel, E., and Baur, R. (1988): *J. Neurosci.*, 8:289-295.
19. Smart, T.G., Houamed, K., von Renterghem, C., and Constanti, A. (1987): *Biochem. Soc. Trans.*, 15:117-122.
20. Stephenson, F.A. (1980): *Biochem. J.*, 249:21-32.

GABA and Benzodiazepine Receptor Subtypes,
edited by Giovanni Biggio and Erminio Costa.
Raven Press, New York © 1990.

ISOLATION OF PHARMACOLOGICALLY DISTINCT

GABA-BENZODIAZEPINE RECEPTORS BY PROTEIN

CHEMISTRY AND MOLECULAR CLONING

R.W. Olsen[1], M. Bureau[1], M. Khrestchatisky[2],
A.J. MacLennan[2], M.-Y. Chiang[2], A.J. Tobin[2], W. Xu[2],
M. Jackson[2], C. Sternini[3], N. Brecha[4]

Departments of Pharmacology[1], Biology[2], Medicine[3], and
Anatomy[4], and Brain Research Institute, University of
California, Los Angeles, CA 90024 USA

The $GABA_A$ receptor is a ligand-gated chloride ion channel
that mediates the majority of rapid-timescale inhibitory
synapses in the central nervous system (3, 39). $GABA_A$
receptors in some and possibly all cellular locations are
subject to pharmacological modulation by both excitatory and
depressant drugs showing a variety of psychiatric and
neurological effects on the brain. The convulsant bicuculline
acts as a GABA receptor antagonist, while picrotoxin and cage
convulsants inhibit the chloride channel function at a site on
the receptor complex distinct from the GABA recognition site
(34). Clinically important depressant drugs including the
benzodiazepines, the barbiturates, the steroid anesthetics, and
possibly ethanol, enhance GABA-mediated inhibition at separate
drug receptor sites directly on the postsynaptic receptor-
chloride ion channel complex (2, 53, 61).

The subject of this symposium was the question of whether
all $GABA_A$ receptors are the same and, in particular, whether
they vary in their pharmacological specificity, especially
sensitivity to the clinically important modulators such as
benzodiazepines. Following a brief introduction on the history
of heterogeneity of GABA-benzodiazepine receptors, we will
present our recent evidence for multiple $GABA_A$ receptor
subtypes based on both protein chemistry and molecular cloning
studies.

35

BRIEF HISTORY OF $GABA_A$ RECEPTOR HETEROGENEITY

GABA synapses and $GABA_A$ receptors are wide-spread and densely situated throughout the nervous system; there is some evidence for pharmacological heterogeneity with tissue (e.g., 1, 15, 18, 33), including variable sensitivity to benzodiazepines (e.g., 41, 43). Radioligand binding studies also suggest heterogeneity for GABA binding (33, 35), benzodiazepine binding (4, 54), and allosteric interactions between the various component receptors on the complex (22, 43, 55, 60, 62). Certain benzodiazepine ligands demonstrated multiple affinities and the subpopulations distinguished by these agents showed a differential distribution and other properties. This included two subpopulations of benzodiazepine binding sites distinguished by high affinity (Type I) or low affinity (Type II) for triazolopyridazines such as CL 218,872 (54), which differ in ontogeny (24) and regional distribution (67). Types I and II should not be equated with the subpopulations distinguished by high affinity (BZ_1) or low affinity (BZ_2) for β-carbolines such as β-carboline-3-carboxylate alkyl esters (4). Although the distribution of these subpopulations has some similarities, e.g., the cerebellum is highly enriched in Type I and BZ_1 receptor binding compared to Type II and BZ_2 (50, 54, 67), the populations defined by triazolopyridazines and β-carbolines do not coincide exactly, since they vary in allosteric interactions with the GABA and barbiturate receptor sites on the complex (22, 32). Brain regional variation in allosteric properties required <u>at least three</u> subpopulations of benzodiazepine receptors. It was speculated that some populations of the complex might not contain all the receptor site components on the complex (22), e.g., some GABA receptors might not have benzodiazepine sites (62), some benzodiazepine receptors might not have GABA sites (24), or the receptor complexes could at least vary in sensitivity to benzodiazepine agonists compared to inverse agonists (see, e.g., chapter by Slobodyansky & Guidotti, this volume).

Binding studies, especially using tissue sections and quantitative autoradiography, showed that Type I and Type II receptors had a differential brain regional distribution (67). Quantitative autoradiography also demonstrated clearly that benzodiazepine and GABA receptor binding did not correspond (66). Muscimol binding showed a higher density in some regions than benzodiazepine binding, e.g., cerebellar granule cell layer and some thalamic nuclei; the density of GABA binding in cerebellar homogenates had been shown to be greater than that of benzodiazepine binding (29). Benzodiazepine binding appeared higher than muscimol in several regions, e.g., substantia nigra, hippocampus, and globus pallidus (66). On the other hand, benzodiazepine binding was enhanced by GABA in all regions to roughly the same extent, indicating that all benzodiazepine receptors were coupled to GABA receptors but not all GABA receptors were coupled to benzodiazepine receptors (62). But radioactive muscimol did not appear to label all of the GABA receptors that participated in enhancement of benzodiazepine binding. This probably was due to the fact that the autoradiography technique, like filtration binding assays, involves a rinse step that dissociates low affinity binding, such that only high affinity (slowly dissociating) binding is detectable (35, 37, 62, 64, 66). The muscimol binding detected using autoradiography has a Kd of about 15 nM (37, 40, 66), while the concentration needed to enhance benzodiazepine binding is micromolar, a concentration closer to that needed for functional activation of chloride channels (2, 61, 62, 64). The question then arises as to whether the high affinity muscimol binding represents a <u>different conformational state</u> of the same receptor protein that is involved in enhancement of benzodiazepine binding (one gene product) or whether <u>different receptor proteins</u> (gene family) are involved.

Different agonist affinity states do exist for the GABA$_A$ receptor, which is an allosteric membrane protein (9) whose activity is mediated by conformational changes (ion channel opening and closing) regulated by ligand binding (34, 39, 64). An antagonist preferring state or type of GABA$_A$ receptor can be detected with radioactive antagonist binding (bicuculline methochloride or SR-95531) and shows micromolar affinities for agonists (27, 30, 38). Nevertheless, the distribution of antagonist (bicuculline) binding does not agree with that of agonist (muscimol) binding and corresponds better with that of benzodiazepine binding (38). On the other hand, attempts to measure intermediate-to-low affinity muscimol binding by autoradiography did not change significantly the distribution of agonist binding, i.e., it still did not agree with antagonist or benzodiazepine binding (37, 40, 62). Indeed, closer examination of seven ligands for the three receptor sites on the GABA$_A$ receptor complex (37) reveals that comparison of any pair of ligands shows considerable discrepancies in densities of binding across brain regions; this includes comparison of [^{3}H]flunitrazepam, the "BZ$_1$-selective" ligand [^{3}H]2-oxo-quazepam, [^{3}H]muscimol, [^{3}H]bicuculline methochloride, [^{3}H]SR-95531, and two cage convulsants [^{35}S]TBPS and [^{3}H]TBOB. In addition to differences in distribution mentioned for GABA agonists versus antagonists and benzodiazepines, and for BZ$_1$ and BZ$_2$ binding sites, there were significant differences in some brain regions between any pair of the seven including two GABA antagonists and two cage convulsants!

This strongly suggests that subpopulations of receptors exist, and a minimum of four such subtypes are required to explain the data. As summarized in Table 1, four subtypes of $GABA_A$ receptors can be defined by brain regions that favor some ligands and disfavor others (37). Thus, at least four subtypes of $GABA_A$-benzodiazepine receptors with different pharmacological properties are demonstrated by binding data alone. Protein chemistry and molecular cloning studies as described below and in other chapters support this interpretation.

Some evidence for distinct benzodiazepine binding proteins was suggested by polyphasic heat inactivation (55), differential solubilization of two fractions (25), differential ontogeny of Type I and Type II activities (24), and multiple peptide bands on SDS gels (49) following photoaffinity labeling of crude homogenates with [^{3}H]flunitrazepam (28). In addition to the major polypeptide band labeled in all brain region that has a molecular weight (Mr) of 51 kiloDaltons (28), minor species are detected in some brian regions at 53, 55, and 59 kDa (49). Since cerebellum showed only the 51 kDa band and Type I/BZ_1 binding activity, this peptide was proposed to correspond to this receptor subpopulation. Other brain regions contained other peptide bands, especially the 55 kDa band; these regions also demonstrated Type II/BZ_2 binding activity, so the 55 kDa polypeptide was proposed to correspond with this binding activity. Sieghart and colleagues (50) showed that the affinity of the 51 kDa band for CL 218,872 was higher than for the other bands, consistent with the designation of the 51 kDa band as Type I receptor. This group also provided evidence that the different bands were probably distinct protein sequences on the basis of ontogeny (13) and proteolytic peptide mapping (48). It now appears likely that these different photolabeled peptide bands are related to the heterogeneity in binding noted above, as well as to different peptide bands in the isolated receptors (see below) and to different subunit sequences identified by cloning. The 51 kDa band with high affinity for triazolopyridazines and beta-carbolines would appear to correspond to the α_1 clone sequence (23, 46; Seeburg et al., and Möhler et al., chapters in this volume). The Type II/BZ_2 subpopulation would appear to consist of a mixture of other peptide bands and subunit clones.

MULTIPLE $GABA_A$-BENZODIAZEPINE RECEPTOR SUBUNITS IDENTIFIED
BY PROTEIN CHEMISTRY AND PHOTOAFFINITY LABELING

The GABA receptor protein in mammalian brain was solubilized with mild detergent (17) and shown to co-purify with the benzodiazepine receptor (59). Deoxycholate and Triton X-100

TABLE 1. GABA$_A$-BZ RECEPTOR SUBTYPES DEFINED BY AUTORADIOGRAPHIC
REGIONAL COMPARISON OF LIGAND BINDING (Olsen et al., 1989)

TYPE	ENRICHED REGIONS	LIGANDS	
		FAVORED	DISFAVORED
1.	SUBSTANTIA NIGRA CEREBELLUM, MOLECULAR LAYER CORTEX, LAYER IV (PERIAQUEDUCTAL GRAY)	*BZ1 ≥ TBOB ≥ BMC	BZ2 ≥ TBPS ≥ MUS > SR-95531*
2.	DENTATE GYRUS SUPERIOR COLLICULUS CORTEX, LAYERS I - III CA1	*BZ2 ≈ SR-95531	BZ1 ≥ TBOB > TBPS
3.	CEREBELLUM, GRANULE LAYER THALAMUS	MUS > TBPS > BMC	BZ1, SR-95531, TBOB > BZ2
4.	NUCLEUS ACCUMBENS (FOR EXAMPLE; OTHER AREAS INCONSISTENT WITH SUM OF 1-3)	BMC ≈ SR-95531	MUSCIMOL

*Underlined ligands are very specific for the subtype indicated. The binding of seven ligands for the GABA receptor complex was measured on thin sections of frozen-thawed rat brain by semi-quantitative autoradiography. Comparisons made on twenty representative regions showed discrepancies in densities for each pair of ligands, many of which were statistically significant. These discrepancies can be explained by a minimum of four subtypes of receptor showing different binding characteristics.

were effective solubilizers, but full native binding and
allosteric properties could be best solubilized with the
zwitterionic bile salt detergent CHAPS (20, 58).
Benzodiazepine affinity chromatography was employed to purify
the protein from bovine brain, with two major bands observed on
SDS gels: α at 53 kDa and β at 56 kDa (52). The α subunit was
heavily labeled and the β subunit lightly photolabeled with
[3H]flunitrazepam (52). Purification in the detergent CHAPS
led to the same purified subunit composition of two
polypeptides, as well as retention of barbiturate interactions
with the GABA and benzodiazepine binding activities (51).

We described a similar purification from rat brain (56), and
identified the major GABA binding site with [3H]muscimol
photoaffinity labeling as the 57 kDa β subunit (12). This rat
preparation contained the same two polypeptide bands as the cow
receptor, the β and α subunits, plus a third band at 47 kDa
shown to be a breakdown product of β and α, and a fourth band
or doublet about 31 kDa, whose identity remains to be
established. The α and β subunit bands were also recognized on
Western blots (56) by a family of monoclonal antibodies,
developed against partially purified bovine receptor, which had
been shown to immunoprecipitate receptor (45).

Partial protein sequence was obtained by Schofield et al.
(46) from the purified bovine receptor, leading to the cloning
of the bovine α and β subunits, deduction of the amino acid
sequences from the full-length complementary DNA's, and
expression of GABA-regulated chloride channels from the
corresponding two messenger RNA's expressed in frog oocytes.
It is now evident that a family of genes exists for both α (23)
and β subunits (65), as well as other related subunits (42), as
discussed below.

Closer examination of the subunit composition of purified
GABA receptor has revealed microheterogeneity of polypeptide
bands on gels (6, 36). Protein staining of long gradient gels
showed that both α and β subunits from rat, cow, and human
receptor were doublets or triplets, and the microheterogeneity
was also observed with immunostaining; the separated peptide
bands were shown to consist of distinct sequences because they
ran as single bands upon repeat electrophoresis in SDS gels or
in isoeletric focussing, they gave unique amino acid
compositions, and they produced unique proteolysis peptide
fragments on one-dimensional peptide mapping gels (8). Other
groups have recently shown that the heterogeneity of α subunits
apparent in [3H]flunitrazepam photolabeling of crude
homogenates (13) is also detectable in purified receptor from
some tissues, using visualization with both photoaffinity
labeling and Western blotting with antibodies (10, 14, 21, 44,
57).

We reported earlier (7) that both [^{3}H]flunitrazepam and [^{3}H]muscimol give photoaffinity labeling of multiple peaks in purified receptor from cow, rat, and human brain, including apparent cross-labeling. Fig. 1 shows a typical experiment for rat receptor. Part A describes [^{3}H]muscimol photolabeling in the absence (▲) and presence (●) of nonradioactive GABA (0.1 mM). Major incorporation is seen in two bands at 55 and 58 kDa corresponding to the stained doublet that is also recognized by immunoblotting with Dr. Möhler's β subunit-specific monoclonal antibody bd17 (not shown here). Smaller but significant labeling is also observed in a doublet at 51 and 53 kDa, corresponding to two stained bands that are also labeled with the α subunit-specific antibody bd28 (bd24 in cow and human, 45). That is, muscimol not only binds to multiple polypeptide bands, but the peptides labeled appear to include those identified as α subunits on the basis of immunoblotting and photoaffinity labeling with [^{3}H]flunitrazepam. The labeling of this same rat receptor with [^{3}H]flunitrazepam is shown in Fig. 1B (□). There is a shoulder at 53 kDa on the major peak at 51 kDa. At higher protein concentrations, lower but significant incorporation of [^{3}H]flunitrazepam into the "β" doublet was observed (7), suggesting that all of the subunits carry both GABA and benzodiazepine binding sites, perhaps with differing affinities.

The different polypeptide bands seen on gels do indeed derive from native receptor oligomers showing different pharmacological properties. When photolabeling was performed in the presence of varying concentrations of nonradioactive receptor ligands, the different bands showed a differential sensitivity to inhibition of photolabeling. For example, different concentrations of the GABA analog 4,5,6,7 tetrahydroisoxazolo-[5,4,c]pyridin-3-ol (THIP) were required to inhibit muscimol binding. In Fig. 1A (O), THIP (0.3 μM) inhibited by over 50% the labeling into the 58 kDa band, but almost insignificantly the labeling of the 56 kDa band; the IC_{50} values for THIP were about 0.2 μM and 3 μM for the 58 and 56 kDa bands, respectively. Likewise, these two bands varied in affinity for muscimol, GABA, and bicuculline, and in their sensitivity to enhancement by barbiturates and anesthetic steroids (Bureau & Olsen, manuscript in preparation). The benzodiazepine binding likewise varied in pharmacological specificity. The 51 kDa band showed a higher affinity than the 53 kDa band for the "Type II"-specific ligand CL 218,872 (8), as seen in crude brain (50). As shown in Fig. 1B (♦), the 53 kDa polypeptide was more sensitive than the 51 kDa band to enhancement by GABA (10 μM), as well as to other allosteric ligands.

The different binding affinities for these multiple distinct polypeptides strongly suggest that purified receptor

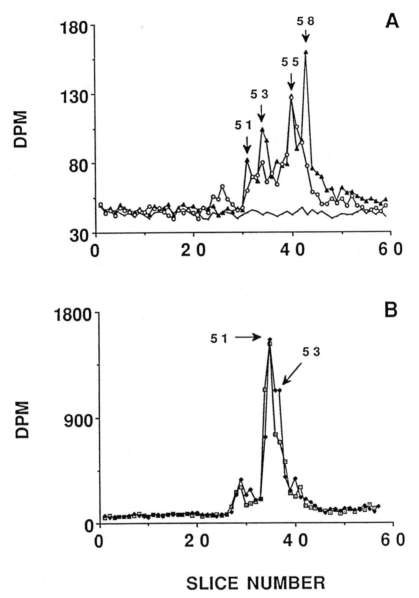

FIG. 1. Photoaffinity labeling of affinity column-purified rat
cortex GABA-benzodiazepine receptor. Samples were run on
SDS-PAGE, sliced (each fraction is 1 mm) and counted for radioactivity. The numbers with arrows represent the Mr determined
from standards in another lane. A. [^{3}H]Muscimol photolabeling
as in (7, 8, 12). No additions (▲); 0.3 μM THIP (O); 0.1 mM
GABA (●). B. [^{3}H]Flunitrazepam photolabeling as in (7, 8, 56).
No additions (□); 10 μM GABA (♦).

preparations actually contain more than one receptor subytpe with different amino acid sequences for the subunits and different pharmacological properties for the oligomers that they form *in vivo*. This conclusion is further supported by observations that this subunit pattern varies with tissue and species. While two major α bands are observed in cerebral cortex receptor, only one band (51 kDa) is isolated from cerebellum, and at least one additional [³H]flunitrazepam labeled band is found in the hippocampus at 55 kDa (8). Likewise, while several mammalian species show a major α band at 51 kDa and tissue-dependent additional bands, the codfish brain shows only a single photolabeled band at 57 kDa that appears to correspond with a single stained band that is also photolabeled with [³H]muscimol. The gene for the codfish receptor peptide may be closely related to the ancestral gene which has evolved into the complex family of subunits seen in mammals (11).

The multiple subunits in mammalian receptor isolated by protein chemistry are thus highly likely to correspond to the multiple genes being isolated. The different binding activities of these isolated proteins provide evidence for distinct receptor subtypes that is complementary to and perhaps even more convincing than studies on "in vitro" expression of cloned genes. It is likely that these receptor subtypes will show differential physiological functions, sensitivity to pathological perturbations, and mechanisms of biological regulation. Preliminary studies (5) indicate that the 56 and 58 kDa β subunits show differential phosphorylation *in vitro* by protein kinases A and C.

NOVEL GABA RECEPTOR SUBUNITS ISOLATED BY MOLECULAR CLONING

Following the initial cloning of the α and β subunits of bovine receptor based on partial protein sequence (46), additional highly similar but different clones were isolated using the original cDNA's as probes. Three distinct α sequences were isolated from cow (23), and one or more of these was also found in human (16, 31) and rat (26, 47). Three distinct β clones have now been sequenced for rat and cow (26, 65), and additional subunits called γ (42) and perhaps others with homologous but distinct sequences have been described (Seeburg et al., Möhler et al., chapters in this volume). The third type of subunit γ may be part of the native oligomeric structure required for full native biological properties of the complex (42). These multiple clones have a differential expression in the nervous system based on Northern blots and *in situ* hybridization (23, 26, 31, 42, 47, 63, 65).

Our group at UCLA (19) has used the published bovine α_1 and β_1 sequences for oligonucleotide hybridization selection of a bovine library to isolate similar cDNA's. These were employed to screen a rat hippocampal cDNA library and three α and two β cDNA's were isolated. Full-length cDNA's were sequenced and an open reading frame including initiation codon was found for each, from which the amino acid sequences could be deduced. One of the α clones is distinct (70% identity) from the previously published three bovine α clones (23) and our other rat α clones, so we have designated it α_4. In Table 2, we compare the properties and expression characteristics of α_4 with the rat α_1 subunit clone, which we found to be nearly identical to the bovine α_1.

Both α_1 and α_4 share sequence motifs common to previously described ligand-gated channel polypeptides (GABA receptors, nicotinic acetylcholine receptors, and the strychnine-sensitive glycine receptor). These include four putative membrane-spanning domains with highly conserved sequences, a long N-terminal presumed extracellular segment containing potential N-glycosylation sites and a conserved cysteine pair believed to participate in forming a ligand-binding site, and a variable region between putative membrane-spanning regions 3 and 4 believed to participate in intracellular regulatory mechanisms. All of the GABA receptor subunits and the other ligand-gated ion channels are considered to share a common evolutionary origin (23, 46).

The deduced rat α_1 sequence contains 428 amino acids plus a signal peptide of 27; there are three residue differences from bovine α_1 in the signal peptide and only one different amino acid in the coding sequence. Rat α_1 shows 76% and 70% identity with cow α_2 and α_3. Rat α_4 contains 433 amino acid residues plus a signal peptide of 31. It shows 70%, 71%, and 66% identity with cow α_1, α_2, and α_3, respectively, with unevenly distributed differences as mentioned.

The presence of α_1 and α_4 messenger RNA in brain was demonstrated by Northern blot and *in situ* hybridization. Poly (A)+ RNA from the frontal cortex showed two distinct mRNA species for α_1 with lengths of 3.8 and 4.3 kb and a single mRNA for α_4 of 2.8 kb. The cerebral cortex, substantia nigra, and hippocampus contained both α_1 and α_4, while the cerebellum contained no α_4 and the striatum contained neither. Antisense probes for α_1 hybridized to cells of the cerebral cortex (all layers), the cerebellum (Purkinje, basket, stellate, and granule cells), and hippocampal formation (some cells in pyramidal and molecular layers, as well as dentate granule layer). The α_4 mRNA was detected in virtually all cells of the pyramidal and granule layers of the hippocampal formation, and at a low level in all layers of the cerebral cortex.

TABLE 2. COMPARISON OF RAT ALPHA$_1$ AND ALPHA$_4$ cDNA's

Sequence	α_1	α_4
Number of amino acids	428	433
Leader sequence	27	31
Identity with bovine α_1, α_2, α_3 (in amino acids)	99,76,70	70,71,66

Messenger RNA

	α_1	α_4
Sizes (kb)	3.8, 4.3	2.8
Distribution		
Hippocampus	++	++
Cerebral cortex	+++	+
Cerebellum	+++	-
Striatum	-	-
Substantia nigra	++	$\pm$

Expression in oocytes

	α_1	α_4
GABA currents	+	+
EC$_{50}$ (μM)	$\approx$5	$\approx$5
Average maximal responses (nA) (to 50 μM GABA)	284	80
Sensitive to picrotoxin	+	+
Picrotoxin currents	+	++

Both α_1 and α_4 cDNA were transcribed *in vitro* and their RNA injected into Xenopus oocytes along with RNA transcribed from a rat β_1-subunit cDNA. After 3-4 days, both gave GABA-activated inward currents consistent with the expression of receptor-ion channels. The half-maximal response to GABA occurred at roughly 5 μM, with maximal responses at 50 μM, but the size of the response was greater for α_1 (plus β) than α_4 (plus β) at all concentrations of GABA. However, this could be due to differential efficiency of translation or protein processing. Picrotoxin reversibly inhibited the response in both cases. Interestingly, picrotoxin alone elicited an outward current in oocytes injected with α_4 plus β, but very rarely with α_1 plus β. We suggest that in the case of α_4 chloride channels, picrotoxin blocks spontaneously opening GABA receptor channels and is actually reducing a tonic inward current. The α_1 and α_4 channels expressed in oocytes thus differ in their responses to both GABA and picrotoxin, although one cannot extrapolate necessarily from the oocyte to the *in vivo* situation in brain neurons (19).

In conclusion, a family of $GABA_A$-benzodiazepine receptor subunits with related gene sequence appears to exist in vertebrate brain and produces a tissue-specific family of receptor subtypes constructed from differing oligomeric combinations of these various subunits. The expression of different genes is likely to involve multiple mechanisms of regulation. The *in vivo* subunit composition remains to be determined, but might be elucidated by a combination of cloning, localization, and protein chemistry. It is important that in addition to the demonstration of different pharmacological properties for different subunit clones expressed *in vitro*, that distinct pharmacological subtypes have been demonstrated to occur in the brain by binding studies and by protein chemistry.

Acknowledgements: Supported by NIH Grants NS22071 and NS21908.

REFERENCES

1. Alger, B.E., and Nicoll, R.A. (1982): *J. Physiol.*, 328:125-141.
2. Biggio, G., and Costa, E., editors (1986): *GABAergic Transmission and Anxiety*. Advances in Biochemical Psychopharmacology, Volume 41. Raven Press, New York.
3. Biggio, G., and Costa, E., editors (1988): *Chloride Channels and Their Modulation by Neurotransmitters and Drugs*. Raven Press, New York.
4. Braestrup, C., and Nielsen, M. (1981): *J. Neurochem.*, 37:333-341.
5. Browning, M.D., Bureau, M., Barnes, E., and Olsen, R.W. (1989): *Abstr. Soc. Neurosci.*, 15:830.
6. Bureau, M., and Olsen, R.W. (1988): *FASEB J.*, 2:A622.
7. Bureau, M., and Olsen, R.W. (1988): *Biochem. Biophys. Res. Comm.*, 153:1006-1011.
8. Bureau, M., and Olsen, R.W. (1989): *Abstr. Soc. Neurosci.*, 15:642.
9. Changeux, J.-P., Devillers-Thiery, A., and Chemouilli, P. (1984): *Science*, 225:1335-1345.
10. de Blas, A.L., and Park, D. (1989): *J. Neurochem.*, 52:S144C (Suppl.).
11. Deng., L., Olsen, R.W., and Nielsen, M. (1988): *Abstr. Soc. Neurosci.*, 14:168.
12. Deng, L., Ransom, R.W., and Olsen, R.W. (1986): *Biochem. Biophys. Res. Comm.*, 1308-1314.
13. Eichinger, A., and Sieghart, W. (1986): *J. Neurochem.*, 46:173-180.

14. Fuchs, K., Möhler, H., and Sieghart, W. (1988): *Neurosci. Lett.*, 90:314-319.
15. Gallagher, J.P., and Shinnick-Gallagher, P. (1983): In: *The GABA Receptors*. edited by S.J. Enna, pp. 25-61. Humana Press, New Jersey.
16. Garrett, K.M., Duman, R.S., Saito, N., Blume, A.J., Vitek, M.P., and Tallman, J.F. (1988): *Biochem. Biophys. Res. Comm.*, 156:1039-1045.
17. Greenlee, D.V., and Olsen, R.W. (1979): *Biochem. Biophys. Res. Comm.*, 88:380-387.
18. Johnston, G.A.R., Allan R.D., and Skerritt, J.H. (1984): In: *Handbook of Neurochemistry*. edited by A. Lajtha, pp. 213-237. Plenum Publishing, New York.
19. Khrestchatisky, M., MacLennan, A.J., Chiang, M.-Y., Xu, W., Jackson, M., Brecha, N., Sternini, K., Olsen, R.W., and Tobin, A.J. (1989) *Neuron*, (in press).
20. King, R.G., Nielsen, M., Stauber, G.B., and Olsen, R.W. (1987): *Eur. J. Biochem.*, 169:555-562.
21. Kirkness, E.F., and Turner, A.J. (1988): *Biochem. J.*, 256:291-294.
22. Leeb-Lundberg, L.M.F., and Olsen, R.W. (1983): *Mol. Pharmacol.*, 23:315-325.
23. Levitan, E.S., Schofield, P.R., Burt, D.R., Rhee, L.M., Wisden, W., Köhler, M., Fujita, N., Rodriguez, H.F., Stephenson, F.A., Darlison, M.G., Barnard, E.A., and Seeburg, P.H. (1988): *Nature*, 335:76-79.
24. Lippa, A.S., Beer, B., Sano, M.C., Vogel, R.A., and Meyerson, L.R. (1981): *Life Sci.*, 28:2343-2347.
25. Lo, M.M.S., Strittmatter, S.M., and Snyder, S.H. (1982): *Proc. Natl. Acad. Sci. USA*, 79:680-684.
26. Lolait, S.J., O'Carroll, A.-M., Kusano, K., Muller, J.-M., Brownstein, M.J., and Mahan, L.C. (1989): *FEBS Lett.*, 246:145-148.
27. McCabe, R.T., Wamsley, J.K., Yezuita, J.P., and Olsen, R.W. (1988): *Synapse*, 2:163-173.
28. Möhler, H., Battersby, M.K., and Richards, J.G. (1980): *Proc. Natl. Acad. Sci. USA*, 77:1666-1670.
29. Möhler, H., and Okada, T. (1977): *Science*, 198:849-851.
30. Möhler, H., and Okada, T. (1977): *Nature*, 267:65-67.
31. Montpied, P., Martin, B.M., Cottingham, S.L., Stubblefield, B.K., Ginns, E.I., and Paul, S.M. (1988): *J. Neurochem.*, 51:1651-1654.
32. Niehoff, D.L., Mashal, R.D., and Kuhar, M.J. (1983): *Eur. J. Pharmacol.*, 92:131-134.
33. Nowak, L.M., Young, A.B., and Macdonald, R.L. (1982): *Brain Res.*, 244:155-164.
34. Olsen, R.W. (1982): *Ann. Rev. Pharmacol. Toxicol.*, 22:245-277.
35. Olsen, R.W., Bergman, M.O., Van Ness, P.C., Lummis, S.C., Napias, C., Watkins, A.E., and Greenlee, D.V. (1981): *Mol. Pharmacol.*, 19:217-227.

36. Olsen, R.W., Bureau, M., Ransom, R.W., Deng, L., Dilber, A., Smith, G., Khrestchatisky, M., and Tobin, A.J. (1988): In: *Neuroreceptors and Signal Transduction.* edited by S. Kito, T. Segawa, K. Kuriyama, M. Tohyama, and R.W. Olsen, pp. 1-14. Plenum, New York.
37. Olsen, R.W., McCabe, R.T., and Wamsley, J.K. (1989): *J. Chem. Neuroanat.*, (in press).
38. Olsen, R.W., Snowhill, E.W., and Wamsley, J.K. (1984): *Eur. J. Pharmacol.*, 99:247-248.
39. Olsen, R.W., and Venter, J.C., editors (1986): *Benzodiazepine/GABA Receptors and Chloride Channels: Structural and Functional Properties.* Receptor Biochemistry and Methodology, Volume 5. Alan R. Liss, New York.
40. Pan, H.S., Frey, K.A., Young, A.B., and Penney, J.B. Jr. (1983): *J. Neurosci.*, 3:1189-1198.
41. Polc, P., Bonetti, E.P., Schaffner, R., and Haefely, W. (1982): *Naunyn Schmiedebergs Arch. Pharmacol.*, 321:260-264.
42. Pritchett, D., Sontheimer, H., Shivers, B.D., Ymer, S., Kettenmann, H., Schofield, P.R., and Seeburg, P. (1989): *Nature*, 338:582-585.
43. Santi, M.R., Cox, D.H., and Guidotti, A. (1988): *J. Neurochem.*, 50:1080-1086.
44. Sato, T.N., and Neale, J.H. (1989): *J. Neurochem.*, 52:1114-1122.
45. Schoch, P., Richards, J.G., Häring, P., Takacs, B., Stähli, C., Staehelin, T., Haefely, W., and Möhler, H. (1985): *Nature*, 314:168-171.
46. Schofield, P.R., Darlison, M.G., Fujita, N., Burt, D.R., Stephenson, F.A., Rodriguez, H., Rhee, L.M., Ramachandran, J., Reale, V., Glencorse, T.A., Seeburg, P.H., and Barnard, E.A. (1987): *Nature*, 328:221-227.
47. Séquier, J.M., Richards, J.G., Malherbe, P., Price, G.W., Mathews, S., and Möhler, H. (1988): *Proc. Natl. Acad. Sci. USA*, 85:7815-7819.
48. Sieghart, W., Eichinger, A., and Zezula, J. (1987): *J. Neurochem.*, 48:1109-1114.
49. Sieghart, W., and Karobath, M. (1980): *Nature*, 286:285-287.
50. Sieghart, W., Mayer, A., and Drexler, G. (1983): *Eur. J. Pharmacol.*, 88:291-299.
51. Sigel, E., and Barnard, E.A. (1984): *J. Biol. Chem.*, 259:7219-7223.
52. Sigel, E., Stephenson, F.A., Mamalaki, C., and Barnard, E.A. (1983): *J. Biol. Chem.*, 258:6965-6971.
53. Squires, R.F., editor (1988): *GABA and Benzodiazepine Receptors.* CRC Press, Florida.
54. Squires, R.F., Benson, D.I., Braestrup, C., Coupet, J., Klepner, C.A., Myers, V., and Beer, B. (1979): *Pharmacol. Biochem. Behav.*, 10:825-830.

55. Squires, R.F., and Saederup, R. (1982): *Mol. Pharmacol.*, 22:327-334.
56. Stauber, G.B., Ransom, R.W., Dilber, A.I., and Olsen, R.W. (1987): *Eur. J. Biochem.*, 167:125-133.
57. Stephenson, F.A., Duggan, M.J., and Casalotti, S.O. (1989): *FEBS Lett.*, 243:358-362.
58. Stephenson, F.A., and Olsen, R.W. (1982): *J. Neurochem.*, 39:1579-1586.
59. Stephenson, F.A., Watkins, A.E., and Olsen, R.W. (1982): *Eur. J. Biochem.*, 123:291-298.
60. Supavilai, P., and Karobath, M. (1980): *Eur. J. Pharmacol.*, 64:91-93.
61. Tallman, J.F., and Gallager, D.W. (1985): *Ann. Rev. Neurosci.*, 8:21-44.
62. Unnerstall, J.R., Kuhar, M.J., Niehoff, D.L., and Palacios, J.M. (1981): *J. Pharmacol. Exp. Ther.* 218:797-804.
63. Wisden, W., Morris, B.J., Darlison, M.G., Hunt, S.P., and Barnard, E.A. (1988): *Neuron*, 1:937-947.
64. Yang, J.S., and Olsen, R.W. (1987): *Mol. Pharmacol.*, 32:266-277.
65. Ymer, S., Schofield, P.R., Draguhn, A., Werner, P., Köhler, M., and Seeburg, P.H. (1989): *EMBO J.*, 8:1665-1670.
66. Young, W.S. III, and Kuhar, M.J. (1980): *J. Pharmacol. Exp. Ther.*, 212:337-346.
67. Young, W.S. III, Niehoff, D., Kuhar, M.J., Beer, B., and Lippa, S. (1981): *J. Pharmacol. Exp. Ther.*, 216:425-430.

GABA and Benzodiazepine Receptor Subtypes,
edited by Giovanni Biggio and Erminio Costa.
Raven Press, New York © 1990.

THE ENDOGENOUS ALLOSTERIC MODULATION OF GABA$_A$

RECEPTOR SUBTYPES: A ROLE FOR THE

NEURONAL POSTTRANSLATIONAL PROCESSING PRODUCTS

OF RAT BRAIN DBI

E. Slobodyansky
A. Berkovich
P. Bovolin
C. Wambebe

FIDIA-GEORGETOWN INSTITUTE FOR THE NEUROSCIENCES
3900 RESERVOIR ROAD
WASHINGTON, D.C. 20007

Pharmacological, molecular biological, and molecular electrophysiological studies now suggest the existence of functionally multiple, and probably structurally multiple, GABA$_A$ receptor subtypes. Functionally, GABA$_{A1}$, GABA$_{A2}$, and GABA$_{A3}$ receptor subtypes can be identified (6, 10, 21, 25, 28). Their common feature is the generation of bicuculline-inhibited Cl$^-$ currents following occupancy of the primary transmitter recognition site by GABA or muscimol (10, 25). Diversity among various subtypes lies in the differences of their apparent sensitivity to GABA (7, 25) and in the structural and functional heterogeneity of the allosteric centers modulating the primary transmitter recognition site located on the GABA receptorial domain (17, 18, 22, 29, and Guidotti, this volume). Since the areas of structural diversity of GABA$_A$ receptor subunits are part of the receptor extracellular domain, where both the allosteric modulatory center and GABA recognition sites are located, it is possible that the structural diversity of the subunits includes the allosteric modulatory centers. Hence, this diversity may be of importance in determining functional specificities of GABA$_A$ receptor subtypes. The allosteric center of the GABA$_{A1}$ receptor, preferentially abundant in cerebellum, contains high affinity recognition sites for the anxiolytic and anticonvulsant benzodiazpines (BZs), triazolopyridazines, and imidazopyridines, as well as high affinity sites for the anxiogenic and proconvulsant beta-carboline-3-carboxylate esters (BCs). The allosteric center of the $GABA_{A2}$ receptor virtually lacks high affinity recognition sites for BCs, clonazepam, triazolopyridazines, or imidazopyridines, but expresses high affinity binding sites for a subgroup of anxiolytic BZs such as diazepam, midazolam, and alprazolam. $GABA_{A2}$ receptors are predominantly located in spinal cord, striatum, and adrenal medulla (5, 6, 21, 22, 24, 29). Olfactory bulb neurons have a high density of BZ recognition sites preferentially labeled by the convulsant benzodiazepine 4'-chloro-diazepam (Ro 5-4864) and by an isoquinoline-carboxamide, PK 11195 (4). We have recently observed that a large amount of Ro 5-4864 binding sites are present on the allosteric modulatory center of the $GABA_A$ receptor. Originally these two ligands were believed to bind in brain to a $GABA_A$-uncoupled BZ recognition site located on glial cells. Recently, behavioral, biochemical, and electrophysiological findings have indicated that Ro 5-4864 and PK 11195 may also bind to a BZ recognition site located on neuronal membranes that may function as an allosteric modulatory center of a novel $GABA_A$ receptor subtype (17, 18, 27, 28, 31), termed the $GABA_{A3}$ receptor (6, 20). Perhaps glial cells may contain still another type of $GABA_A$ receptor ($GABA_{A4}$) in which BCs function as positive allosteric modulators (11).

To obtain further evidence in support of the hypothesis that Ro 5-4864 can bind to the allosteric center of the $GABA_{A3}$ receptor, we began an investigation on the cellular and subcellular distribution and molecular nature and function of the allosteric modulatory center that includes Ro 5-4864 binding sites in brain.

Approximately 1/3 of the total Ro 5-4864 binding in brain has been found in synaptic plasma membranes (unpublished observations). The Ro 5-4864 binding sites present on $GABA_A$ receptors have a number of characteristics that allow the differentiation of these sites from those present in mitochondria. We have found that protoporphyrin IX displaces Ro 5-4864 from mitochondria but not from synaptic plasma membranes. On the other hand, TBPS (t-butylbicyclophosphorothionate) and picrotoxinin displace Ro 5-4864 allosterically from synaptic plasma membranes but not from mitochondria. Since picrotoxinin and TBPS bind to a site on the $GABA_A$ receptor different from the BZ site, we have used the allosteric property of picrotoxinin or TBPS as a tool to evaluate the amount of Ro 5-4864 binding sites coupled to $GABA_A$ receptors in different brain areas. Among the investigated regions, the richest in this binding is the olfactory bulb; the lowest are the cortex and the cerebellum (unpublished data).

We further studied the existence of Ro 5-4864 binding at the $GABA_A$ receptor in human tumor embryonic kidney cells (cell line 293) transfected with cDNA encoding for different subunits of the $GABA_A$ receptor. Before transfection these cells have no GABA receptors and a small number of Ro 5-4864 binding sites

(K_D~50nM, Bmax~1 pmol/mg protein). Transfection with alpha$_1$, beta$_1$, and gamma$_2$ subunits of GABA$_A$ receptors leads to the expression of GABA$_A$ receptors and to an increase in the number of Ro 5-4864 binding sites (up to ~3 pmol/mg protein), as well as to a shift in ligand affinity from 50 to ~150nM. However, the binding site of Ro 5-4864 to the newly expressed GABA$_A$ receptor subtype cannot be the flumazenil binding site since ^{3}H-Ro 5-4864 can be displaced by Ro 5-4864 but not flumazenil.

Is diazepam binding inhibitor (DBI) the precursor of neuropeptides that act at different GABA$_A$ receptor subtypes?

A key question raised by the structural and functional heterogeneity of the allosteric modulatory centers of GABA$_A$ receptor subtypes is whether or not each GABA$_A$ receptor subtype is regulated by specific endogenous ligands. DBI is a 10kDa peptide present in rat and human brain (16,19,26); it depresses the GABA-induced Cl$^-$ current in patch-clamped embryonic spinal cord neurons (9, 10) and displaces BZs, BCs, and Ro 5-4864 from their respective binding sites on cultured neurons or astroglial cells (8, 13, 15, 21). These observations, together with the fact that DBI structure includes several basic amino acids that can be sites of proteolytic cleavage (Fig. 1), lead to the proposal that DBI may function as a precursor for a family of biologically active neuropeptides operating as putative endogenous ligands at the different GABA$_A$ receptors (14, 15). Tryptic digestion of rat DBI yields an octadecaneuropeptide, ODN, that includes amino acid residues 33-50 of the DBI sequence. ODN, like DBI, displaces flunitrazepam, BCs, and flumazenil from binding sites on neurons with an affinity of approximately 1uM (15), but unlike DBI it fails to displace Ro 5-4864 (21). When ODN is injected intraventricularly into rats and mice it mimics the anxiogenic action elicited by BCs acting as negative allosteric modulators of the GABA$_A$ receptors (15, 23).

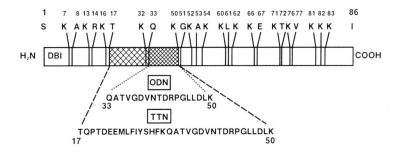

Fig. 1. Amino acid sequence of rat brain DBI (1-86) and its processing products: TTN (DBI 17-50) and ODN (DBI 33-50).

Using polyclonal antibodies raised against synthetic ODN, it was found that brain contains several DBI peptide fragments that immunoreact with these antibodies. This ODN-LI (ODN-like immunoreactivity) is localized in neurons, particularly in GABAergic axon terminals, where it is stored in synaptic vesicles and can be released with the primary transmitter upon depolarization (14, 21).

Two questions are raised by these observations: (1) what is the structure of these ODN-like peptides, and (2) do the ODN-LI peptides released at specific brain synapses function as natural chemical signals endowed with the ability to discriminate among different $GABA_A$ receptor subtypes.

DBI 33-50 (ODN)and DBI 17-50 (Triakontatetraneuropeptide; TTN): two posttranslational processing products of DBI in rat brain

Reverse phase HPLC analyses of brain homogenates from rats killed by microwave irradiation reveal the presence of four major peptide peaks that react with ODN antiserum (Fig. 2).

One of the peaks is presumably DBI itself and expresses the crossreactivity of DBI with ODN-antibodies. Because the amount of DBI-LI present in acetic extract of microwaved rat brain is much higher than the amount of ODN-LI, we separated ODN-LI peptides from DBI-LI peptides by gel-filtration on Bio-Gel P-6. The ODN-LI fractions were then subjected to purification on CNBr-activated Sepharose 4B coupled with ODN-antibodies (30).

The use of immunoaffinity chromatography with ODN-immuno-globulins immobilized on CNBr-activated Sepharose 4B, combined with analytical and microbore reverse phase HPLC steps, shows that the peptide TTN (DBI 17-50) (for the structure characteristics, see Fig. 1) is the most abundant component of the three ODN-LI peaks present in rat brain extracts (30). The other two ODN-LI peaks that emerge from HPLC have also been purified following ODN immunoaffinity chromatography. The first of these two peaks coelutes from the HPLC reverse phase column with ODN, and presumably is ODN itself. The other ODN-LI peak fails to coelute with any of the synthetic peptides we used as reference standards. Since this later peak contains smaller amounts of material, its sequence analysis is, so far, incomplete.

TTN and ODN are the first posttranslational processing products of rat brain DBI that have been isolated and characterized. ODN is an 18 amino-acid peptide obtained previously as the major product of tryptic digestion of DBI; TTN is a 34 amino acid peptide whose sequence corresponds to that of amino acids between DBI positions 17-50. When 3 ug of synthetic TTN was added to an acetic acid brain extract and run through the purification procedure, approximately 2-3% of the peptide was recovered. Taking into account that the affinity of the ODN antibody for TTN is about 10 times weaker than it is for ODN, as estimated by RIA, we calculate that the rat brain content of TTN should be around 100 pmole/mg protein, whereas that of ODN is approximately 5-10 pmol/mg protein.

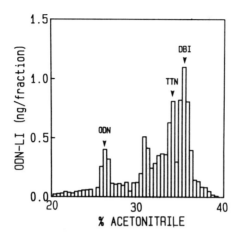

Fig. 2. **Reverse phase HPLC profile of ODN-LI peptides in the acetic acid extract of microwaved rat brain. Arrows indicate the positions of rat DBI and synthetic ODN and TTN (for details see ref. 30).**

TTN includes the amino acid sequence of ODN, plus a chain of 16 amino acids flanking the amino terminus of ODN. A computer-assisted analysis of DBI hydrophobicity spectra indicates that ODN is hydrophilic while, in the TTN sequence, the 16 amino acid chain that extends from the amino terminus of ODN is strongly hydrophobic and capable of assuming an alpha-helical configuration (21); this is an interesting feature of TTN. Since TTN is present in axon terminals (3), its helicity may be important in determining receptorial specificity when it is released from neurons in a Ca^{2+}-dependent manner during depolarization (14).

TTN and ODN distribution and localization in rat brain

As described previously (1, 2), DBI- and ODN-LI were detected in many brain regions. The most intense signals were found in cerebellum, amygdala, reticulothalamic nucleus, hypothalamus, and hippocampus. Using antibodies raised against TTN, we found that the distribution of TTN-LI was similar to that of ODN-LI (3). ODN-LI and TTN-LI were localized in neurons exclusively, whereas DBI-LI was present in neurons and in glia or glial-like cells lacking ODN-LI or TTN-LI. Probably the posttranslational processing of neuronal DBI differs from that in glia (2, 3).

In other brain regions, ODN- and TTN-LI were located in scattered neurons throughout the cerebro-cortical layers. As shown in Fig. 3, a dense network of neurons intensively stained with antibodies is present in the reticulothalamic nucleus.

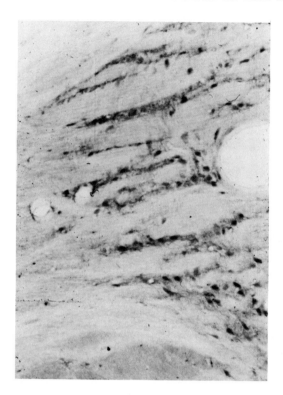

Fig. 3.

TTN-LI in the rat reticular thalamic nucleus: all neurons contain positive immunoreactive material (for details, see ref. 2, 3).

Electronmicroscopically this immunoreactivity appears to be compartmentalized in synaptic vesicles (2). Because there is cross-reactivity between ODN and TTN-antiserum and TTN and ODN-antiserum, monoclonal antibodies directed toward structurally different amino acid sequences of ODN and TTN should be prepared in order to study whether these different DBI processing products are localized in different cell types.

Pharmacology of TTN and ODN

Since TTN and ODN were found to be most abundant among ODN-LI peptides in rat brain, we then focused on the characterization of their pharmacological properties.

Pharmacological, behavioral, and binding data obtained with synthetic TTN provide evidence that this naturally occuring peptide may represent a DBI processing product important for the allosteric modulation of the $GABA_{A3}$ receptor subtype. ODN, in contrast, may be the natural ligand for the $GABA_{A1}$ receptor subtype.

When tested on the punishment-conflict behavioral paradigm described by Corda (12), TTN is at least one order of magnitude more potent than DBI and 4-5 fold more potent than ODN in

inducing conflict behaviour . In this test, TTN is not only more potent than ODN or DBI but is also longer lasting. However, the effect of TTN is not due to its being processed to ODN or to ODN-like peptides because the proconflict action elicited by TTN, unlike that of ODN, is virtually unchanged by pretreatment with flumazenil (Table 1). This inhibitor, which binds with high affinity to the allosteric modulatory center of the $GABA_{A1}$ and $GABA_{A2}$ receptor subtypes (6, 29), completely blocks the proconflict action of ODN and BCs. The proconflict effect of TTN, like that of Ro 5-4864, is blocked by PK 11195, a drug that fails to block the effects of ODN and BCs suggesting an interaction of TTN with Ro 5-4864 binding sites in brain (Table 1).
In line with this conclusion is the finding that ODN, but not TTN, displaces ^{3}H-flumazenil bound to primary cultures of cerebellar granule cells. In contrast, TTN efficiently displaces ^{3}H-Ro 5-4864 bound to astroglial homogenates, while ODN (50 uM) is devoid of such activity (Table 1). Based on our behavioral and displacement studies and on the immunohistochemical detection of TTN in neurons exclusively, we

TABLE I: PHARMACOLOGICAL PROFILE OF ODN AND TTN

PEPTIDE	Binding		Proconflict activity (licking periods/3 min)		
	^{3}H-flumazenil to cerebellar granule cells Ki, uM	^{3}H-Ro 5-4864 to astroglial homogenates Ki, uM	Pretreatment [a]		
			Vehicle	Flumazenil 2mg/kg i.v.	PK 11195 2mg/kg i.v.
NONE	-	-	24 ± 2.0	26 ± 4.2	24 ± 1.8
ODN	1.5 ± 0.22	>50	$7 \pm 1.5^*$	22 ± 4.2	$7 \pm 1.0^*$
TTN	>50	1.0 ± 0.12	$8 \pm 0.7^*$	$12 \pm 1.8^*$	$22 \pm 3.2^*$

[a] Peptides (i.c.v.): 3.0 nmol ODN; 1.0 nmol TTN. Rats received flumazenil or PK-11195 10 min before i.c.v. injection of the indicated peptide. Proconflict activity (12) was measured 5 min after the peptide injection.

* P < 0.001 when compared with saline treated rats.

propose that TTN may function in brain by binding to Ro 5-4864 recognition sites. To investigate further the interaction at the $GABA_A$ receptor between TTN and Ro 5-4864, we studied the binding of ^{3}H-Ro 5-4864 to highly purified synaptosomal membranes prepared from rat olfactory bulb, which are known to include the highest neuronal density of Ro 5-4864 recognition sites. TTN displaces ^{3}H-Ro 5-4864 from its binding sites on olfactory bulb synaptosomal membranes with a potency (K_i~5uM) higher than that of ODN (K_i>100μM). Unlike ODN, which displaces ^{3}H-flunitrazepam (15) or ^{3}H-flumazenil (Table 1) from recognition sites on neuronal membranes, TTN cannot displace these ligands but, similarly to Ro 5-4864, it facilitates picrotoxinin-induced inhibition of GABA-stimulated ^{3}H-flunitrazepam binding. Since the TTN binding profile resembles that of Ro 5-4864, the suggestion that it may act as a negative allosteric modulator of $GABA_{A3}$ receptor subtypes is upheld. TTN also displaces ^{3}H-Ro 5-4864 from binding sites located on astrocytic membranes (Table 1). Thus, it cannot be excluded that the TTN neuropharmacological profile might include actions on the allosteric modulatory center of the GABA-gated Cl^- channels located on astrocytic membranes (11).

CONCLUSIONS

These experiments support the view that DBI may serve as the precursor in brain for smaller biologically active neuropeptides that function as putative negative allosteric modulators of $GABA_A$ receptor-mediated effects. Among these peptides we have positively identified ODN and TTN (see Fig. 1), the latter being the most abundant. TTN-LI, as well ODN-LI, was found exclusively in neurons, and, although both TTN and ODN cause proconflict activity in rats, they obviously produce similar effects by different mechanisms. In fact, in the Vogel conflict test TTN mimics Ro 5-4864 while ODN acts similarly to FG7142, a beta-carboline-3-carboxylate ester derivative. Moreover, TTN displaces ^{3}H-Ro 5-4864, but not ^{3}H-flumazenil, from synaptic membranes with a K_i of approximately 5 uM, while ODN displaces ^{3}H-flumazenil but not ^{3}H-Ro 5-4864. In addition, TTN also enhances picrotoxinin inhibition of GABA-stimulated ^{3}H-flunitrazepam binding. Our present working hypothesis is that TTN and ODN are two putative endogenous allosteric modulators each acting on different $GABA_A$ receptor subtypes.

REFERENCES

1. Alho, H., Costa, E., Ferrero, P., Fujimoto, M., Cosenza-Murphy, D., and Guidotti, A. (1985): *Science*, 229: 179-182.

2. Alho, H., Bovolin, P., Jenkins, D., Guidotti, A. and Costa, E. (1989): *J. Chem. Neuroanatomy*, in press.

3. Alho, H., Bovolin, P. and Slobodyansky (1989): *J. Neurochem. Res.*, in press.

4. Anholt, R.R.H., De Souza, E.B., Oster-Granite, M.L. and Snyder, S.H. (1985): *J. Pharmacol. Exp. Ther.*, 233: 517-526.

5. Arbilla, S., Allen, J., Wick, A. and Langer, S.Z. (1986): *Eur. J. Pharmac.*, 130: 257-263.

6. Barbaccia, M.L., Costa, E., and Guidotti, A. (1988): *Annual Rev. Pharmacol. Toxicol.*, 28: 451-476.

7. Barnard, E.A., Burt, D.R., Darlison, M.G., Fujita, N., Levitan, E.S., Schofield, P.R., Seeburg, P.H., Squire, M.D. and Stephenson, F.A. (1989): In: *Allosteric modulation of amino acid receptors: Therapeutic Implications*, E.A. Barnard and E. Costa eds., pp.19-30 Raven Press, New York.

8. Bender, A.S. and Hertz, L. (1986): *Eur. J. Pharmacol.*, 132: 335-336.

9. Bormann, J., Ferrero, P., Guidotti, A. and Costa, E.: (1985) *Regulatory Peptides*, 264: 33-38.

10. Bormann, J. (1988): *TINS*, 11: 112-116.

11. Bormann, J. and Kettenmann, H. (1988): *Proc. Natl. Acad. Sci. USA*, 85: 9336-9340.

12. Corda, M.G., Blocker, W.D., Mendelson, W.B., Guidotti, A. and Costa, E. (1983): *Proc. Natl. Acad. Sci USA*, 80: 2072-2076.

13. Costa, E., Berkovich, A. and Guidotti, A. (1987): *Life Sci.*, 41: 799-803.

14. Ferrarese, C., Alho, H., Guidotti, A. and Costa, E.: (1987) *Neuropharmacology*, 26: 1011-1018 .

15. Ferrero, P., Santi, M.R., Conti-Tronconi, B., Costa, E. and Guidotti, A. (1986): *Proc. Natl. Acad. Sci. U.S.A.*, 83: 827-831.

16. Ferrero, P., Costa, E., Conti-Tronconi, B. and Guidotti, A. (1986): *Brain Res.*, 399: 136-142.

17. Gee, K.W. (1986): *J. Pharmacol. Exp. Ther.*, 240: 747-753.

18. Gee, K.W., Brinton, R.E. and McEven, B.S. (1987): *J. Pharmacol. Exp. Ther.*, 244: 379-383.

19. Guidotti, A., Forchetti, C.M., Corda, M.G., Konkel, D., Bennett, C.D., and Costa, E. (1983): *Proc. Natl. Acad. Sci. U.S.A.*, 80: 3531-3535.

20. Guidotti, A., Berkovich, A., Ferrarese, C., Santi, M.R. and Costa, E. (1988): In: *Imidazopyridines in Sleep Disorders*, J.P. Sauvanet, S.Z., Langer, and P.L. Morselli, eds., pp. 25-38 Raven Press, New York.

21. Guidotti, A., Alho, H., Berkovich., A., Cox, D.H., Ferrarese, C., Slobodyansky, E., Santi, M.R. and Wambebe, C. (1989): In: *Allosteric modulation of amino acid receptors: Therapeutic implications*, E.A. Barnard and E. Costa, eds., pp. 100-123 Raven Press, New York.

22. Kataoka, Y., Gutman, Y., Guidotti, A., Pauela, P., Wroblewski, J., Cosenza-Murphy, D., Wu, J.Y. and Costa, E. (1984): *Proc. Natl. Acad. Sci. U.S.A.*, 81: 3218-3222.

23. Kavaliers, M, and Hirst, M. (1986): *Brain Res.*, 383: 343-349.

24. Klepner, C.A., Lippa, A.J., Benson, D.I., Santo, M.C. and Beer, B. (1979): *Pharmacol. Biochem. and Behav.*, 11: 457-462.

25. Levitan, E.S., Schofield, P.R., Burt, D.R., Rhee, L.M., Wisden, W., Kohler, M., Fujita, N., Rodriguez, H.F., Stephenson, A., Darlison, M.G., Barnard, E.A. and Seeburg, P.H. (1988): *Nature*, 335: 76-79.

26. Marquardt, H., Todaro, G.J. and Shoyab, M. (1986): *J. Biol. Chem.*, 2261: 9727-9731.

27. Mizoule, J., Gauthier, A., Uzan, A., Renault, C., Dubroeucq, M.C., Gueremy, C. and Le Fur, G. (1985): *Life Sci.*, 36: 1059-1068.

28. Puia, G., Santi, M.R., Vicini, S., Pritchett, D.B., Seeburg, P.H. and Costa, E. (1989): *PNAS*, in press.

29. Santi, M.R., Cox, D.H., Guidotti, A. (1988): *J. Neurochem.*, 50: 1080-1086.

30. Slobodyansky, E., Guidotti, A., Wambebe, C., Berkovich, A. and Costa, E. (1989): *J. Neurochem.*, in press.

31. Weissman, B.A., Cott, J., Hommer, D., Quirion, R., Paul, S., Skolnick, P. (1983): *Benzodiazepine Recognition site ligands: Biochemistry and Pharmacology*, G. Biggio, and E. Costa eds. pp. 139-151 Raven Press, New York.

GABA and Benzodiazepine Receptor Subtypes,
edited by Giovanni Biggio and Erminio Costa.
Raven Press, New York © 1990.

ZOLPIDEM AND ALPIDEM: TWO IMIDAZOPYRIDINES WITH SELECTIVITY FOR ω_1- AND ω_3-RECEPTOR SUBTYPES

S.Z. Langer, S. Arbilla, J. Benavides and B. Scatton

Department of Biology,
Synthélabo Recherche (L.E.R.S.),
58, rue de la Glacière, 75013 Paris, France

Zolpidem and alpidem are imidazopyridine (Fig. 1) derivatives possessing preferential affinities for omega receptor subtypes in both animals and man. Zolpidem is a hypnoselective agent while alpidem is a non-sedative anxiolytic (2,9,10,18,23). The recent development of drugs possessing only some of the pharmacological actions of benzodiazepines (hypnotic, muscle relaxant, anticonvulsant and anxiolytic) has reinforced the concept of the existence of ω-receptor subtypes (1,2,4,14,24) at which these drugs may interact to exert their preferential pharmacological actions. The nomenclature of these receptors corresponds to a pharmacological criterion based on the variety of chemical structures with selective affinities for the three receptor subtypes. Receptors of the ω_1 type correspond to those identified by agonists such as the triazolopyridazine, CL 218872, inverse agonists such as the ß-carboline ß-CCE and the antagonist pyrazoloquinolinone CGS 8216 (11-13). The ω_2-receptor is recognized in a non-selective manner by agonists possessing a benzodiazepine structure, or by the antagonist imidazodiazepine flumazenil (11-13). Finally, the ω_3-receptor corresponds to the peripheral type, which recognizes selectively the benzodiazepine Ro 5-4864 or the isoquinoline carboxamide PK 11195 (11-13). Here, we demonstrate that omega receptor subtypes can also be identified with imidazopyridines such as zolpidem or alpidem which possess different pharmacological and therapeutic profiles.

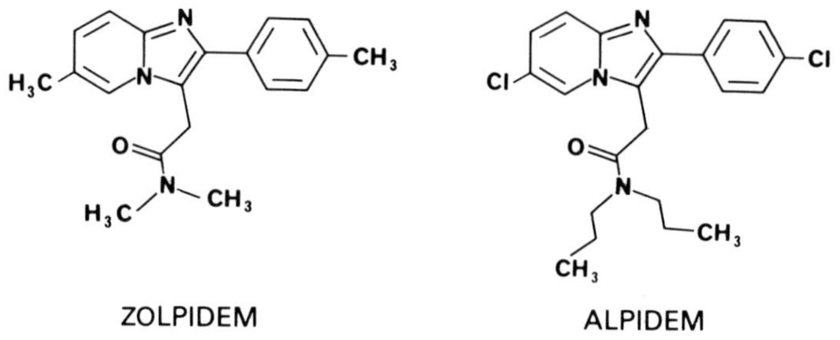

ZOLPIDEM   ALPIDEM

FIG. 1. Chemical structures of the imidazopyridines zolpidem and alpidem

INTERACTION OF ZOLPIDEM AND ALPIDEM WITH OMEGA RECEPTORS LABELLED WITH BENZODIAZEPINES

The cerebellum, spinal cord and kidneys are examples of tissues that possess predominantly receptors of the ω_1, ω_2 and ω_3 type, respectively (19,24,25). It is now well established that the majority of benzodiazepines lack selectivity for ω-receptor subtypes. Consequently, the selectivity of a drug for ω-receptor subtypes is evaluated in studies of displacement of benzodiazepine binding to tissues differentially enriched in a given ω-receptor subtype. The relative potencies and the selectivity of zolpidem and alpidem for ω_1-, ω_2- and ω_3-receptor subtypes labelled with [3H]-flumazenil or [3H]-Ro 5-4864 are shown in table 1. The imidazopyridine zolpidem possesses preferential affinity for the ω_1-site in the cerebellum when compared with its affinity for the ω_2-site in the spinal cord (Table 1). Alpidem also possesses a higher affinity for ω_1-sites than for ω_2-sites. It has to be mentioned as well that in autoradiographic studies performed in the rat (19) and in the monkey (J. Benavides and B. Scatton, unpublished results) brain, the selectivity ratio of alpidem for ω_1- as compared to ω_2-sites ranged from 2.8 to 6 and was much lower than that of zolpidem. In contrast with zolpidem, alpidem has a very high affinity for ω_3-sites labelled with [3H]-Ro 5-4864 in the kidney (Table 1). The receptor binding profile of the preferential ω_1-receptor partial agonist, the triazolopyridazine CL 218872 is shown for comparison (Table 1).

TABLE 1. Relative potencies of zolpidem and alpidem to displace [^{3}H]-flumazenil and [^{3}H]-Ro 5-4864 binding to membrane preparations from rat tissues containing different ω-receptor subtypes

Compounds	IC_{50} (nM)			
	[^{3}H]-FLU Cerebellum	[^{3}H]-FLU Spinal cord	[^{3}H]-Ro 5-4864 Kidney	ω_2/ω_1
	ω_1-site	ω_2-site	ω_3-site	ratio
Zolpidem	14	130	1,900	9.3
Alpidem	18	76	0.9	4.2
CL 218872	73	440	> 10,000	6

Drug concentrations inhibiting binding by 50% were obtained from inhibition curves derived from at least 8 concentrations of each drug tested. Shown IC_{50} values are means of at least 2 independent experiments carried out in duplicate. FLU: flumazenil.

The selectivity of zolpidem for ω_1-receptors was more pronounced when studied in the primate brain. As shown in table 2, zolpidem was 73-fold more potent at displacing [^{3}H]-flunitrazepam binding from ω_1-receptors in the cerebellum than from ω_2-receptors in the dentate gyrus in the monkey. In this species, CL 218872 (Table 2) also shows higher selectivity for ω_1-receptors than in the rat (Table 2).

TABLE 2. Relative potencies of zolpidem to displace [^{3}H]-flunitrazepam binding to regions containing different ω-receptors in coronal sections of monkey brain

	IC_{50} (nM)		
	Cerebellum (ω_1-site)	Dentate gyrus (ω_2-site)	ω_2/ω_1 ratio
Zolpidem	5.5	400	72.7
CL 218872	70	900	12.9
Flumazenil	4.5	4.5	1

TABLE 2 (cont.)
Brain sections were incubated with 1 nM [^{3}H]-flunitrazepam in the presence of 1 μM PK 11195 and five or six concentrations of the displacing drug. Non-specific binding was defined by 2 μM flumazenil and subtracted from all density values. Data for IC_{50} determinations were mean values of eight density readings per region from 2 monkeys as described by Dennis et al. (8).

BINDING CHARACTERISTICS OF IMIDAZOPYRIDINES AT OMEGA RECEPTOR SUBTYPES

Studies of high affinity binding of either zolpidem or alpidem were performed in membranes from different tissues using both imidazopyridines in their tritiated form. Zolpidem as radioligand was shown to bind in central tissues to a single population of recognition sites (1,12,13). In the rat, [^{3}H]-zolpidem possesses similar affinity for its recognition site in the cerebral cortex and the cerebellum (Table 3). From the differences in the density of [^{3}H]-zolpidem binding sites measured in different tissues, it is likely that the recognition site for [^{3}H]-zolpidem belongs exclusively to the ω_1-type. As shown in table 3, the spinal cord does not possess detectable levels of [^{3}H]-zolpidem binding. The pharmacological profile of [^{3}H]zolpidem binding confirms the ω_1-selectivity of this compound.

Under conditions in which specific binding either to ω_1/ω_2-receptors or ω_3-receptors is appropriately defined (12), [^{3}H]-alpidem can be shown to bind to a single population of non-interacting sites. The existence of a binding site of ω_2-type in the rat cerebral cortex can be excluded because binding to these receptors does not occur in the spinal cord (Table 3). In addition to the affinity of [^{3}H]-alpidem for ω_1-sites, the compound possesses high affinity for ω_3-sites in cortex (Table 3). The affinity of [^{3}H]-alpidem for ω_3-sites is, as it was expected from [^{3}H]-benzodiazepine binding competition data (Table 1), much higher than the one for ω_1-receptors (Table 3).

IDENTIFICATION OF ω_1-RECEPTOR DISTRIBUTION IN THE MONKEY BRAIN USING [^{3}H]-ZOLPIDEM AS A SELECTIVE LIGAND

Due to the marked selectivity of zolpidem for ω_1-receptors in the brain of the monkey, as measured by its capacity to displace [^{3}H]-flunitrazepam binding (Table 2), [^{3}H]-zolpidem represents a ligand of choice to identify the regional distribution of ω_1-receptors in the primate central nervous system. As shown in table 4, the quantitative autoradiographic distribution of [^{3}H]-zolpidem binding sites in the monkey brain is compatible with the known distribution of ω_1- and ω_2-receptors in the rat and mouse central nervous system (3,19). Preferential enrichment in ω_1-sites

TABLE 3. Binding characteristics of [3H]-zolpidem and [3H]-alpidem to ω-receptors in membranes from rat brain and spinal cord

Central	Site	[3H]-ALPIDEM		[3H]-ZOLPIDEM	
		K_d (nM)	B_{max} (fmol/mg prot)	K_d (nM)	B_{max} (fmol/mg prot)
Cerebellum	ω_1	7.20 ± 0.50	1100 ± 70	0.82 ± 0.06	783 ± 51
Cortex	ω_1/ω_2	7.10 ± 0.50	1700 ± 60	1.50 ± 0.14	1440 ± 129
Cortex	ω_3	N.T.	N.T.	0.033 ± 0.003	189 ± 8
Spinal cord	ω_2	(-)	(-)	(-)	(-)

The dissociation constant (K_d) and the maximal number of binding sites (B_{max}) were calculated from linear Scatchard plots of saturation analysis. Specific [3H]-zolpidem binding to ω-receptors in different tissues was measured as described by Arbilla et al. (1). Specific [3H]-alpidem binding to ω_1/ω_2-sites in central tissues defined in the presence of flumazenil 2 µM was determined in membranes preincubated for 10 min with PK 11195 2 µM. Binding of [3H]-alpidem to ω_3-sites was determined as described by Langer and Arbilla (12). The data are means $\pm$ S.E.M. of at least 3 individual determinations. (-): not detectable. N.T.: not tested.

TABLE 4. Comparative autoradiographic analysis of [3H]-zolpidem and [3H]-flunitrazepam binding to ω-receptors in the monkey brain

Brain region	fmol/mg prot			Ratio $\dfrac{\omega_1}{\omega_1 + \omega_2}$
	[3H]-Flunitrazepam ($\omega_1 + \omega_2$)	[3H]-Zolpidem (ω_1)	[3H]-Flunitrazepam + zolpidem (ω_2)	
Gyrus frontalis (level 1) I-III	755 ± 23	250 ± 17	319 ± 10	0.33
IV	1111 ± 19	581 ± 28	372 ± 10	0.52
V-VI	792 ± 19	322 ± 21	303 ± 12	0.40
Gyrus frontalis (level 2) I-III	908 ± 29	318 ± 8	290 ± 15	0.35
IV	1329 ± 36	673 ± 24	318 ± 14	0.54
V-VI	918 ± 29	337 ± 10	239 ± 10	0.36
Caudate nucleus matrix	512 ± 15	76 ± 13	246 ± 8	0.15
patches	744 ± 30	234 ± 20	356 ± 16	0.31
Nucleus accumbens	736 ± 45	94 ± 19	363 ± 20	0.13
Globus pallidus p. med.	509 ± 31	283 ± 28	79 ± 11	0.56
p. lat.	527 ± 27	277 ± 31	83 ± 11	0.53
Amygdala (entire complex)	890 ± 48	197 ± 17	451 ± 15	0.22
Dentate gyrus molecular layer	1642 ± 110	191 ± 17	829 ± 53	0.12
granular layer	716 ± 36	74 ± 12	376 ± 23	0.10
Cerebellum molecular layer	545 ± 22	341 ± 20	100 ± 13	0.63
granular layer	738 ± 55	462 ± 22	73 ± 8	0.63

Coronal sections were incubated as described by Dennis et al. (8) with 5 nM [3H]-zolpidem or 1 nM [3H]-flunitrazepam in the presence of 1 μM PK 11195. For displacement determinations, adjacent tissue sections were incubated with 1 nM [3H]-flunitrazepam in the presence of 1 μM PK 11195 and 100 nM zolpidem. Non specific binding determined by incubation of adjacent tissue sections in the presence of 2 μM Ro 15-1788 was subtracted from all density readings. Levels 1 and 2 refer to Brodman areas 9 and 6. Results are means ± S.E.M. of 8 readings per region from 3 monkeys.

was detected in the cerebral cortex, particularly layer IV; globus pallidus, substantia nigra and cerebellum (Table 4; Ref. 8). On the other hand, ω_2-receptors are predominant in the dentate gyrus, caudate nucleus, nucleus accumbens and amygdala (Table 4).

DIFFERENCES BETWEEN IMIDAZOPYRIDINES IN THEIR ACTIVITY AT THE ω_1-GABA RECEPTOR CHLORIDE CHANNEL MACROMOLECULAR COMPLEX

The GABA$_A$ receptor that includes the chloride-ionophore and the picrotoxin-barbiturate site is known to be associated with the ω-receptor (5,6,15,20). The binding of both imidazopyridines, [3H]-alpidem and [3H]-zolpidem involves an ω-receptor associated with the GABA$_A$ receptor since it is increased in the presence of GABA (Table 5), confirming the agonist properties of both compounds at their recognition site. The effect of GABA on [3H]-zolpidem binding has been shown to be associated with an increase in the affinity for its recognition site (1).

TABLE 5. Influence of GABA, chloride ions and pentobarbital on [3H]-imidazopyridine binding to ω_1-receptors in the rat cerebral cortex

	% enhancement		
	GABA (10 μM)	Cl$^-$ (100 mM)	Pentobarbital (1 mM)
[3H]-Zolpidem	117 ± 18*	51 ± 6*	30 ± 5*
[3H]-Alpidem	82 ± 12*	11 ± 5	2 ± 4

Specific binding at a single concentration of [3H]-zolpidem (2 nM) and [3H]-alpidem (1 nM) was determined in the absence (controls) or in the presence of GABA, Cl$^-$ions or pentobarbital at the concentration indicated within parentheses. The experimental conditions used are described by Arbilla et al. (1). Data are expressed as the percent changes in the specific binding relative to the control values and represent the means ± S.E.M. of 3 to 5 experiments carried out in duplicate. * p < 0.05 when compared with control values.

Chloride ions at 100 mM produce an increase in the binding of [3H]-zolpidem (Table 5) but do not affect the binding of [3H]-alpidem (Table 5). Under our experimental conditions, this increase in [3H]-zolpidem binding by chloride ions is statistically significant although rather modest when compared with the 90% increase produced by chloride ions in the binding of a benzodiazepine like diazepam (1). It was suggested that the chloride-ionophore is associated preferentially with the ω_2-receptor (15). Therefore, the modest effect of chloride ions on the binding of the two imidazopyridines may be related to the preferential action of zolpidem and alpidem at ω_1-receptors. Alternatively, this poor sensitivity to chloride may reveal the existence of subtile differences between the imidazopyridine and benzodiazepine interaction with ω_{1-2}-binding sites. Pentobarbital, which enhances the binding of benzodiazepines, also facilitated the binding of [^{3}H]-zolpidem (Table 5). As shown in table 5, pentobarbital was inactive on [^{3}H]-alpidem binding.

DISCUSSION

In contrast to benzodiazepines which in general possess low selectivity for omega receptor subtypes, the two imidazo-pyridines, alpidem and zolpidem possess considerable selectivity for omega receptor subtypes. Both compounds have a preferential affinity for the ω_1- as compared to the ω_2-receptor. In addition, there is a marked difference between alpidem and zolpidem regarding their selectivity for the ω_3-receptor. Zolpidem has very low affinity for the ω_3-receptor, while alpidem is at present the compound with the highest affinity for this receptor subtype.

The selectivity of zolpidem for ω_1-receptors was first demonstrated in rat brain membranes. Similar selectivity of zolpidem for ω_1-receptors was also reported in sections of both rat and mouse brain (3,19). The autoradiographic study of the regional selectivity of zolpidem at displacing [^{3}H]-flunitrazepam binding in the monkey brain sections indicates that zolpidem is a more selective ligand for ω_1-receptors in the monkey than in rodents. In fact, the selectivity of zolpidem for ω_1- as compared to ω_2-receptors was 73-fold in the monkey brain and about 7-fold in rodents. The comparative autoradiographic analysis of [^{3}H]-zolpidem and [^{3}H]-flunitrazepam binding densities in the monkey brain indicates that ω_1-sites in this species are predominantly located in sensorimotor structures while ω_2-sites are essentially present in the limbic system. Thus, zolpidem appears as the ligand of choice to identify and characterize ω_1-sites in the primate brain.

The receptor binding data in rat cerebral cortex membranes indicate that alpidem, similarly to zolpidem, behaves as an agonist with respect to its allosteric interaction with the $GABA_A$ receptor. In fact, GABA increases the binding of alpidem as well as zolpidem and this effect is considered as an index of the intrinsic activity of a compound (17). An increase in the affinity of a ligand either by ions that penetrate the chloride ionophore (7,16) or by barbiturates which interact at a specific site in the chloride channels (21) might also reflect the intrinsic activity of a compound. In contrast to zolpidem, the binding of alpidem is not affected by the presence of either chloride ions or pentobarbital.

Thus, the binding of zolpidem is sensitive to conformational changes in the ω_1-receptor elicited allosterically through the recognition sites for GABA or barbiturates as well as at the chloride channel level (Fig. 2). On the other hand, alpidem binding is only sensitive to the allosteric interactions mediated via the GABA recognition site in the $GABA_A$ receptor complex. This particular profile is perhaps indicative of a low intrinsic activity in the facilitation of the opening of the chloride channel and may relate to the weak sedative potential of alpidem (27). Yet, GABA increases [3H]-alpidem and [3H]-zolpidem binding to an almost similar extent. In contrast to alpidem, zolpidem behaves as a full agonist leading to a hypnotic activity.

RESTING STATE

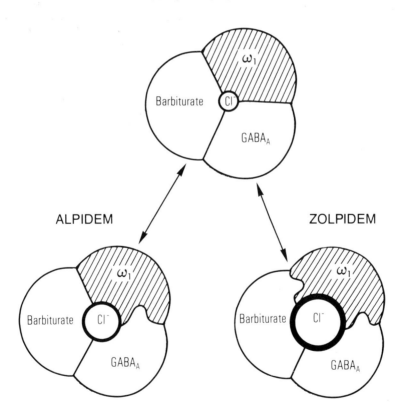

FIG. 2. Model for ω_1-receptor function

The pharmacological effects of the activation of the ω_1-site are thought to occur at the level of a macromolecular complex consisting of a chloride channel, a barbiturate receptor, a $GABA_A$ recognition site and an ω_1-receptor. In the absence of ligands (resting state), the frequency of the opening of the chloride channel is low. The ω_1-receptor activation may result in conformational changes in $GABA_A$ receptor complex. Alpidem binding to the $GABA_A$ receptor complex is sensitive to the degree of occupancy of the GABA binding site while zolpidem binding is also sensitive to the occupancy of the barbiturate site. The degree of activation of the chloride ionophore (shown schematically as the diameter of the central circle) by a particular ω_1-ligand may be related to these allosteric interactions.

The affinity of alpidem for ω_3-receptors in the rat tissues is very high, representing the drug with the highest affinity for ω_3-receptors available. Although there is no conclusive evidence in favor of the efficacy of a selective ω_3-ligand in the treatment of anxiety, it is tempting to speculate on the possible involvement of ω_3-receptors in this disorder. The density of ω_3-receptors is reduced in platelets of anxious patients (26) and beneficial effects of the selective ligand for ω_3-receptors, PK 11195 appear to occur in patients with anxious or depressive symptomatology (22).

At present, the functional and pharmacological relevance of omega receptor subtypes remains an open question. The availability of drugs such as the two imidazopyridines alpidem and zolpidem, which differ from each other and from classical benzodiazepines, in their profile of receptor subtype selectivity as well as the level of their interaction with GABA receptor macromolecular complex may provide useful tools to study this problem.

REFERENCES

1. Arbilla, S., Allen, J., Wick, A., and Langer, S.Z. (1986): Eur. J. Pharmacol., 130:257-263.

2. Arbilla, S., Depoortere, H., George, P., and Langer, S.Z. (1985): Naunyn-Schmiedeberg's Arch. Pharmacol., 330:248-251.

3. Benavides, J., Peny, B., Dubois, A., Perrault, G., Morel E., Zivkovic, B., and Scatton, B. (1988): J. Pharmacol. Exp. Ther., 245:1033-1041.

4. Braestrup, C., and Nielsen, M. (1981): J. Neurochem., 37: 333-341.

5. Briley, M., and Langer, S.Z. (1978): Eur. J. Pharmacol., 52: 129-132.

6. Costa, E., Guidotti, A., and Toffano, G. (1978): Br. J.

Psychiat., 133:239-245.

7. Costa, T., Rodbard, D., and Pert, C.B. (1979): Nature, 277: 315-317.

8. Dennis, T., Dubois, A., Benavides, J., and Scatton, B. (1988): J. Pharmacol. Exp. Ther., 247:309-322.

9. Depoortere, H., Zivkovic, B., Lloyd, K.G., Sanger, D., Perrault G., Langer, S.Z., and Bartholini, G. (1986): J. Pharmacol. Exp. Ther., 237:649-658.

10. Desager, J.P., Hulhoven, R., Harvengt, C., Hermann, P., Guillet, P., and Thiercellin, J.F. (1988): Psychopharmacology, 96:63-66.

11. Langer, S.Z., and Arbilla, S. (1987): 5th Int. Congress of Sleep Research, Abst 050.

12. Langer, S.Z., and Arbilla, S. (1988a): Pharmacol. Biochem. Behav., 29:763-766.

13. Langer, S.Z., and Arbilla, S. (1988b): Fundam. Clin. Pharmacol., 2:159-170.

14. Le Fur, G., Guilloux, F., Rufat, P., Benavidès, J., Uzan, A., Renanet, C., Dubroeucq, C., and Gueremy, C. (1983): Life Sci. 32:1849-1856.

15. Lo, M.M.S., and Snyder, S.H. (1983): J. Neurochem., 11: 2270-2275.

16. Martin, I.L., and Candy, J.M. (1980): Neuropharmacology, 19: 1175-179.

17. Möhler, H., and Richards, J.G. (1981): Nature, 294:763-765.

18. Nicholson, A.N., and Pascoe, D.A. (1986): Br. J. Pharmacol., 21:205-211.

19. Niddam, R., Dubois, A., Scatton, B., Arbilla ,S., and Langer, S.Z. (1987): J. Neurochem., 49:890-899.

20. Olsen, R.W. (1981): J. Neurochem., 31:1-6.

21. Olsen, R.W. (1982): Ann. Rev. Pharmacol. Toxicol., 22: 245-277.

22. Papart, P., Anssean, M., Cerfontaine, J.C., and von Frenckell R. (1988): Psychopharmacology, 96 (Suppl): Abst 28.33.11.

23. Saletu, B., Grunberger, J., and Linzmayer, L. (1986): Int. J. Clin. Psychopharmac., 1:145-164.

24. Schoemaker, H., Boles, R.G., Horst, W.D., and Yamamura, H.I. (1983): J. Pharmacol. Exp. Ther., 225:61-69.

25. Watanabe, Y., Khatami, T., Shibuya, T., and Salafsky, B. (1985): Eur. J. Pharmacol., 109:307-310.

26. Weizmann, R., Tanne, Z., Granek, M., Karp, L., Golomb, M., Tyano, S., and Gavish, M. (1987): Eur. J. Pharmacol., 138:289-292.

27. Zivkovic, B., Morel, E., Joly, D., Perrault, G., Sanger, D.J., and Lloyd, K.G. (1989): Pharmacopsychiatry (in press).

Acknowledgements
The authors are grateful to Miss Françoise Péchoux for preparing the manuscript.

GABA and Benzodiazepine Receptor Subtypes,
edited by Giovanni Biggio and Erminio Costa.
Raven Press, New York © 1990.

THE DIFFERENCES IN THE PHARMACOLOGICAL PROFILES OF VARIOUS BENZODIAZEPINE RECOGNITION SITE LIGANDS MAY BE ASSOCIATED WITH GABA$_A$ RECEPTOR STRUCTURAL DIVERSITY

GUIDOTTI, A., ANTONACCI, M.D., GIUSTI, P., MASSOTTI, M. [*]
MEMO, M. and SCHLICHTING, J.L.

FIDIA-GEORGETOWN INSTITUTE FOR THE NEUROSCIENCES
SUITE SE-402
3900 RESERVOIR ROAD, N.W.
WASHINGTON, D.C. 20007

[*]LABORATORIO DI FARMACOLOGIA
ISTITUTO SUPERIORE DI SANITA
00161 ROMA, ITALY

ALLOSTERIC INTERACTIONS AT THE GABA$_A$ RECEPTOR AS A BASIS FOR HETEROGENEITY

Multiple chemical signals (primary transmitters, cotransmitters, and modulators) which interact at a given receptor domain to contribute increased or decreased synaptic strength may help to explain individual diversity of higher brain functions and may be used for improving specific targeting of neuroactive drugs (10). Functional domains of a number of synaptic receptors may include multiple recognition sites for primary transmitters and allosteric modulators which participate in the transmission of information exchange at synapses (4, 10, 14). The multiple recognition sites associated with a given receptor domain can interact with each other to bring about positive and negative cooperativity in the allosteric modulation of primary transmitter-mediated receptor function (10). Often the intrinsic activity of an allosteric modulator depends on the availability of the primary neurotransmitter at the specific receptor site. The allosteric modulator by binding to its recognition site can change the probability of receptor responsiveness to the primary neurotransmitter. Thus, synaptic strength can be modulated by the interactions of two signals,

which makes the intensity of the response in part independent
from the amount of primary transmitter released by the nerve
terminal. A classical example of allosteric modulation at CNS
synapses is the change in the probability of $GABA_A$ receptor
response to GABA induced by several neuropharmacologically
important classes of drugs, such as benzodiazepines (BZs) and
beta carboline-3-carboxylate esters (BCs) (4, 10, 13, 14). It
is possible their negative and positive allosteric modulatory
action mimics endocoids present in the brain (i.e., DBI and its
processing products or BZ-like molecules, endogenously present
in the mammalian brain) (13, 18). Classically, the best
described form of the $GABA_A$ receptor includes on its domain,
in addition to recognition sites for $GABA_A$, an allosteric
modulatory center which contains recognition sites for the
classical anxiolytic BZs and the anxiogenic BCs (12, 14).
Although the exact stoichiometry of this receptor domain is as
yet uncertain, the $GABA_A$ receptor complex is known to be a
heteropolymeric structural protein which spans the neuronal
membrane and includes at least two alpha and two beta subunits.
The receptor, in addition to alpha and beta subunits possibly
includes gamma and delta subunits, approximately similar in
molecular weight (50 kDa) and with abundant structural homology,
which may confer structural and functional diversity to the
receptor (4, 25, 20).
In mammalian central and peripheral nervous tissues $GABA_A$
receptor diversity has been inferred even before the
documentation of structural differences. In fact, binding and
pharmacological profiles of BZs have suggested the existence of
several subclasses of $GABA_A$ receptors (13). The $GABA_A$
receptor subclasses include a diversity of allosteric modulatory
centers as reflected by specific BZ binding profiles. For
example, $GABA_{A1}$ and $GABA_{A2}$ receptor subclasses have been
defined by the presence of two subtypes of BZ binding sites on
the $GABA_A$ receptor domain, one with high affinity for the
anxiolytic BZs, BCs, CL 218,872 and zolpidem (BZ1 subtype), and
one with high affinity for anxiolytic BZs such as diazepam and
flunitrazepam and low affinity for BCs, clonazepam, zolpidem, or
CL 218,872 (BZ2 subtype) (3, 7, 15, 16, 22). Recently, a third
$GABA_A$ receptor subclass, the $GABA_{A3}$ receptor, has been
demonstrated in the brain and shown to be associated with BZ
binding sites which recognize Ro 5-4864 (4'Cl-diazepam) and PK
11195 (isoquiniline carboxamide) (12, 21, Slobodyansky, this
volume). Thus, within the $GABA_A$ receptor complex, the
allosteric modulatory center which binds BZs and BCs, or
4'Cl-diazepam or PK 11195 exhibits heterogeneity.
Binding, photoaffinity labelling and structural studies suggest
heterogeneity of the $GABA_A$ receptor complex. For instance,
BCs displace flunitrazepam from the cerebellar synaptic
membranes with an apparent higher affinity than that found in
the hippocampus (7). Furthermore, the B_{max} of ^{3}H-PrCC
(^{3}H-propyl-beta-carboline-3-carboxylate) is only 57% and 71%

that of ^{3}H-flunitrazepam in the rat hippocampus and in the rat cerebral cortex respectively, whereas the B_{max} of ^{3}H-PrCC is identical to ^{3}H-flunitrazepam's in the rat cerebellum (7).   In addition, the allosteric modulatory centers of GABA$_A$ receptors which are located in the rat spinal cord and cow adrenal medulla bind flumazenil, diazepam, and flunitrazepam, but are virtually unable to bind anxiogenic BCs or zolpidem (3, 15, 21, 23). Heterogeneity of the allosteric modulatory center has also been inferred from photoaffinity labelling studies with flunitrazepam.   When saturating concentrations of flunitrazepam are bound to brain synaptic membranes in the presence of u.v. irradiation, the ligand binds irreversibly to the BZ sites. In such photolabelled membranes, virtually deprived of ^{3}H-BZ binding capability, ^{3}H-BCs continue to bind reversibly at the original B_{max} (27).   Recent studies on the structural characteristics of GABA$_A$ receptors suggest the different subclasses of GABA$_A$ receptors identified by BZ binding studies may have a discrete heterogeneity in the amino acid sequence of the protein subunits which contribute to the formation of the allosteric modulatory center.   The following experimental evidence supports the above hypothesis: A)   In the adrenal medulla and the spinal cord, where the allosteric modulatory center of the GABA$_A$ receptor complex fails to bind BCs, zolpidem, and CL 218,872, the physicochemical characteristics of

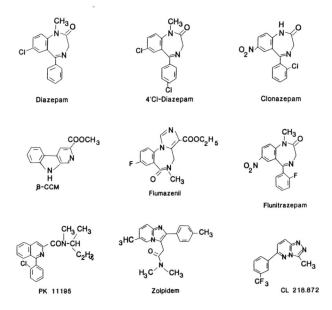

Figure 1.   Chemical structures of BZ ligands which recognize different allosteric modulatory sites on the GABA$_A$ receptor domain.

the subunits which contribute to the function of the receptor appear to be different from those found in the cerebellum (24); B) In situ hybridization studies conducted with oligonucleotide probes for the different alpha, beta, gamma and delta subunits of the GABA$_A$ receptor reveal discrete distribution of the multiple subunits in those brain areas which also show heterogeneity of BZ binding (17, 26, 28). C) Electrophysiological (6) and molecular cloning experiments (20) have revealed the existence of a GABA$_A$ receptor subtype on glial cell membranes which is positively modulated by BZs and BCs and contains a subunit composition different from that present in neurons. Thus the data support the existence of a multiplicity of GABA$_A$ receptor subtypes.

BENZODIAZEPINE LIGAND BINDING HETEROGENEITY PROVIDES EVIDENCE FOR THE EXISTENCE OF GABA$_A$RECEPTOR SUBTYPES

The existence in the mammalian CNS of GABA$_A$ receptor subclasses which are structurally heterogeneous, preferentially located in strategic CNS structures, and characterized by BZ binding site heterogeneity might help to explain the distinct pharmacological profile of several chemically related BZ binding site ligands. To verify these working hypotheses we have

TABLE 1:   BINDING OF VARIOUS LABELLED BENZODIAZEPINE
LIGANDS TO CRUDE SYNAPTIC MEMBRANES OF RAT CNS

CNS Region	DIAZEPAM	CLONAZEPAM	ZOLPIDEM	FLUMAZENIL	BETA-CCM
	B_{max} (pmol/mg prot)				
Olfactory bulb	2.2	2.3	2.0	2.2	–
Cortex	2.0	2.2	1.8	2.0	–
Cerebellum	1.8	2.1	1.3	1.8	1.8
Striatum	1.6	0.95	0.42	1.6	–
Spinal cord	0.9	0.1	<0.1	0.85	<0.1

B_{max} values obtained from saturation iosotherms of ^{3}H-diazepam, ^{3}H-clonazepam, ^{3}H-zolpidem, ^{3}H-flumazenil and ^{3}H-beta-CCM binding to membranes prepared from various rat CNS areas. K_D values are as follows: Diazepam (15-20 nM); Clonazepam (1.5-2.3 nM); Zolpidem (7-9 nM); Flumazenil (1-3 nM) and beta-CCM (5-8 nM).

compared the pharmacological profile of diazepam, zolpidem, clonazepam, and beta carboline-3-carboxylate methyl ester (beta-CCM) with their binding characteristics in different areas of rat CNS.

The binding charcteristics of clonazepam were compared with those of diazepam (a BZ known to bind equally well at BZ recognition sites associated with all GABA$_A$ receptor subtypes throughout the CNS) (23), with flumazenil (a BZ modulator antagonist which binds to GABA$_{A1}$ and GABA$_{A2}$ receptor subtypes) (23), and with those of zolpidem and beta-CCM (drugs known to bind to the GABA$_{A1}$ receptor subtypes in the cerebellum and cortex, but not to the GABA$_{A2}$ receptor subtypes in the spinal cord or the other brain areas) (3, 23).

Clonazepam has been portrayed as the ideal ligand for "central" BZ recognition sites (8, 14). However, extensive binding studies using clonazepam have not been reported in the literature. Clonazepam is known to have a peculiar pharmacological and clinical profile, and although structurally very similar to diazepam (see Fig. 1) it differs from diazepam pharmacologically because: a) it does not bind to peripheral BZ binding site (8), b) it behaves as a partial agonist in several pharmacological and electrophysiological tests (5, 11), c) it elicits less sedation than diazepam (5), and d) it has an anticonvulsant profile more suitable to clinical applications than diazepam (19). Hence we decided to examine ^{3}H-clonazepam binding to different CNS areas to assess whether the pharmacological and clinical profile of this drug can be explained by the presence of a heterogeneous population of binding sites in the CNS. Uniformly labelled ^{3}H-clonazepam (80 Ci/mM), HPLC purified, was obtained as a generous gift from Hoffmann LaRoche (Nutley, NJ); and binding isotherms to crude synaptic membranes from the different CNS regions were analyzed using standard procedures.

The results of these studies (Table 1) demonstrate high affinity (K_D~2 nM) and high capacity (approximately 2 pmol/mg prot) binding of ^{3}H-clonazepam to crude synaptic membranes obtained from rat cerebellum, cortex, and olfactory bulb. In these brain areas the density of ^{3}H-clonazepam binding sites is similar to that labelled by ^{3}H-diazepam, ^{3}H-zolpidem, ^{3}H-flumazenil, and ^{3}H-beta -CCM (Table 1). In contrast, in the striatum, the number of binding sites for ^{3}H-clonazepam is significantly less than for ^{3}H-diazepam or ^{3}H-flumazenil. In the spinal cord, the high affinity binding for ^{3}H-clonazepam is at the limit of detection (Bmax below 0. 1pmol/mg prot), whereas the density of high affinity binding for ^{3}H-diazepam and ^{3}H-flumazenil is approximately 1/2 the density of high affinity sites found in the cerebellum (approximately 2 pmol/mg prot) (Table 1).

The pattern of distribution for ^{3}H-clonazepam binding in the different brain areas is qualitatively similar to that for the

^{3}H-beta-CCM and ^{3}H-zolpidem. However, the density of ^{3}H-zolpidem binding sites in the striatum is less than that of clonazepam (approximately 1/2).

The potency of diazepam or flumazenil in displacing ^{3}H-flumazenil bound to spinal cord and cerebellar membranes was similar (Table 2). In contrast, clonazepam, like zolpidem, CL 218-872, and beta-CCM displaces ^{3}H-flumazenil, which is bound to cerebellar membranes at a potency 10- to 100- fold stronger than that required to displace ^{3}H-flumazenil from the spinal cord membranes. Table 2 shows the IC_{50} values derived from concentration-dependent displacement curves using as ligands 1 nM ^{3}H-flumazenil for the cerebellar membranes and the spinal cord membranes or 1 nM ^{3}H-clonazepam in the cerebellum, only. ^{3}H-clonazepam displacement curves in the

TABLE 2:   DISPLACEMENT OF ^{3}H-FLUNITRAZEPAM
^{3}H-CLONAZEPAM BOUND TO CRUDE SYNAPTIC MEMBRANES
OF RAT CEREBELLUM AND SPINAL CORD

	CEREBELLUM				SPINAL CORD	
	^{3}H Flunitrazepam		^{3}H Clonazepam		^{3}H Flunitrazepam	
DISPLACING DRUG	IC_{50} (nM)	n_H	IC_{50} (nM)	n_H	IC_{50} (nM)	n_H
Diazepam	20 ± 3.0	1.0	18 ± 3.0	1.0	26 ± 3.2	1.0
Flumazenil	1.0 ± 0.080	1.0	1.0 ± 0.010	0.90	1.9 ± 0.10	0.95
Clonazepam	0.85 ± 0.03	1.1	0.75 ± 0.10	0.98	50	<0.5
Zolpidem	10 ± 0.92	0.95	10 ± 2.0	0.90	100	<0.5
CL 218,872	12 ± 0.080	0.90	15 ± 0.09	1.2	>100	<0.5
beta-CCM	1.4 ± 0.20	0.95	1.5 ± 0.03	0.90	60 ± 2.5	<0.5
Ro 5-4864	>1000	-	>1000	-	>1000	-
PK 11195	>1000	-	>1000	-	>1000	-

Each value represents the mean inhibitor concentration (IC_{50}) +/- standard error obtained from displacement dose-response curves. The values are results of at least three different experiments.

^{3}H-Flunitrazepam 1nM, ^{3}H-Clonazepam 1nM; n_H = Hill number.

spinal cord were not reported because, as shown in Table 1, ^{3}H-clonazepam exhibits only a low binding to the spinal cord at this concentration. Table 2 also shows Hill coefficients for the displacing agents. The Hill coefficient approaches 1 in cerebellar membranes for all ligands studied, whereas, in spinal cord, clonazepam, zolpidem, CL218,872, and beta-CCM have Hill coefficients lower than 0.5, indicating a non-isosteric interaction or the existence of multiple binding sites. Neither 4'Cl-diazepam nor PK 11195, two ligands for GABA$_{A3}$ receptor subtype (see Table 4), was capable of displacing ^{3}H-flunitrazepam or ^{3}H-clonazepam at concentrations up to 10^{-6}M (Table 2). This data suggests that in addition to the classical GABA$_A$ receptor prototype in the CNS which expresses an equal number of BZ and BC recognition sites, there exist structurally different GABA$_A$ receptors which do not contain recognition sites for BCs, zolpidem, or clonazepam. Perhaps every brain area has a different proportional representation of

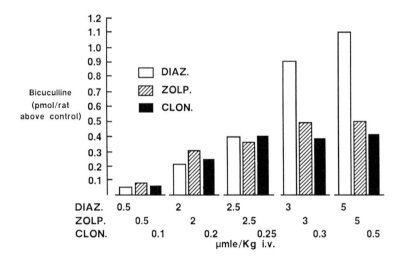

Figure 2. Dose relationship between diazepam, clonazepam or zolpidem and bicullulline seizure test. Rats received i.v. infusion of biculluline solution (0.27 umol/ml) at a rate of 0.46 ml/min. The infusion was stopped after the first full myoclonic convulsion. Normal control rats convulsed within the first 2-3 min (delivered volume of approximately 0.8-1.3 ml).

the various GABA$_A$ receptor subtypes which in turn may differ in the structure of the allosteric modulatory center.

PHARMACOLOGICAL EVIDENCE FOR GABA$_A$ RECEPTOR HETEROGENEITY

As previously discussed (23) diazepam binds with equal potency at benzodiazepine recognition sites associated with all GABA$_A$ receptor subtypes throughout the CNS (see Table 2). If clonazepam and zolpidem, however, recognize BZ recognition sites associated with particular GABA$_A$ receptor subtypes which are found most abundantly in cortical and cerebellar regions (i.e., not those associated with the GABA$_A$ receptor subtypes, in the spinal cord, or the striatum) then the pharmacological profile of diazepam would be expected to differ from that of clonazepam and zolpidem.

To evaluate the pharmacological action of various BZs on the GABA$_A$ receptor function in vivo, relevant data can be obtained by quantifying the convulsant action of bicuculline (a selective GABA$_A$ recognition site isosteric antagonist) in the presence or absence of BZ treatment (9).

The bicuculline seizure test consists of giving a slow infusion of (+)- bicuculline into the tail vein of the rat and recording the time required to elicit the first signs of myoclonus as well as the onset of full myoclonic convulsions (see Fig. 2 for details).

This reasoning prompted us to compare the effect of diazepam, clonazepam, and zolpidem on bicuculline-induced convulsions and on intrinsic ability to induce ataxia and motility changes.

Diazepam and zolpidem increased the seizure latency at doses several-fold higher than doses of clonazepam (Fig. 2). This was expected based on binding studies which demonstrated clonazepam has an affinity for the BZ binding sites at least 10-fold higher than diazepam and 5-fold higher than zolpidem. However, these studies also revealed the efficacy of clonazepam and zolpidem in the bicuculline test differs from diazepam. Doses of clonazepam (0.3 to 2.0 umol/kg) and zolpidem (0.25 to 5 umol/kg) which reached similar maximal levels of protection to bicuculline-induced seizure did so at an apparent maximal efficacy which was found to be significantly less than the efficacy of diazepam (see Fig 2). When comparing doses of clonazepam, zolpidem, and diazepam, which had equipotent effects in the bicuculline seizure test to tests which assess ataxia and motor function we found clonazepam caused significantly less effect on the motility score when compared to diazepam and zolpidem and virtually no effect on the wire test and ataxia scores when compared to saline-treated controls (see table 3).

In summary, the results from the various paradigms used to compare diazepam, clonazepam, and zolpidem suggest a correlation between the lack of binding of clonazepam and zolpidem in the spinal cord and the striatum to their marked lack of effects on ataxia at doses which are equipotent with diazepam in the bicuculline seizure test. Interestingly, in the bicuculline test clonazepam and zolpidem were significantly less efficacious than

TABLE 3: RAT BEHAVIORAL RESPONSES TO ACUTE
BENZODIAZEPINE TREATMENT

ACUTE TREATMENT	MOTILITY RATE (Counts per 3 min)	WIRE TEST (score)	ATAXIA (score)
Saline	830 $\pm$ 56	0	0
Diazepam 2.7 umol/Kg	150 $\pm$ 9.5	+++	2-3
Zolpidem 2.5 umol/Kg	120 $\pm$ 8	+	0-1
Clonazepam 0.3 umol/Kg	480 $\pm$ 89	+	0-1

Drug naive rats received a single intravenous injection of saline, diazepam, clonazepam, or zolpidem and were assessed for their responses in three separate tests within five minutes of the injection time. Each sample group consisted of 8-12 rats. The table represents results from one of three similar experiments. Motility rates represent the mean +/- SEM. Wire test scale: (+++) rats fall when suspended from wire, (++) rats remain suspended with their front paws, (+) rats lift at least one hind paw to the wire. Ataxia scoring scale: 1) mild ataxia; 2) gross ataxia; 3) inability to stand with trunk off table; 4) loss of righting reflex.

diazepam (see Fig 2). However, the difference in efficacy cannot be explained by differences in drug metabolism (this lab, unpublished) and therefore implies an involvement of different GABA$_A$ receptor subtypes.
If clonazepam has action at a subpopulation of BZ recognition sites associated with a GABA$_A$ receptor subtype predominantly present in the cerebellum and the cerebral cortex but not in the spinal cord, and biculluline is antagonizing GABA at all the GABA$_A$ receptor subtypes, a plateau of clonazepam protective response to the biculluline seizure test would not be unexpected. On the other hand, diazepam which has positive modulatory effects at all GABA$_A$ receptors described including those present in spinal cord (see Tables 1 and 2) would show a higher intrinsic efficacy for protecting against seizures induced by biculluline infusion.
While clonazepam is considered a "central" type BZ recognition site ligand with greater potency than diazepam (8), binding

experiments have shown the two BZs have different regional binding distribution in brain. That clonazepam does not bind to high affinity sites in the spinal cord and recognizes a different number of binding sites in the striatum, suggests the action of clonazepam may be mediated through a subpopulation of the total number of recognition sites to which BZs, like diazepam, bind and elicit their actions. While the concept of clonazepam as a partial agonist (5, 11, 14) is a reasonable one, it is not supported by the results of binding studies, which have shown the number of sites recognized by diazepam or clonazepam differs considerably. Clearly, the frequently asserted view that BZ ligands all have the same profile of action since they interact with the same receptor is no longer tenable. It is important to note, the BZ recognition site ligand, zolpidem, which like clonazepam produces anticonvulsant (Fig. 2) and anticonflict effects (22), induces minor ataxic effects (see Table 3) yet fails to bind to spinal cord membranes (Table 1). Moreover, zolpidem also differs from clonazepam because it not only recognizes a smaller number of binding sites in the striatum, but also possesses a strong sedative action (see motility score, Table 3) which is absent at equivalent anti-convulsant doses of clonazepam. In conclusion, these experiments suggest the ataxic effects of diazepam are related to action at GABA$_A$ receptor subtypes in the spinal cord, while sedative effects common to both diazepam and zolpidem may result from action at GABA$_A$ receptor subtypes such as those recognized by zolpidem in the striatum.

CLASSIFICATION OF GABA$_A$ RECEPTOR SUBTYPES

Table 4 lists a provisional classification of GABA$_A$ receptor subtypes as defined by the binding characteristics of ligands to the allosteric modulatory center. At least 5 different subclasses of BZ binding sites can be identified from our studies in the GABA$_A$ receptor domain. In agreement with previous reports (3, 7 ,16, 23), the BZ1 site has high affinity for the anxiolytic BZ clonazepam, the triazolopiridazine CL 218,872, the imidazopyridine zolpidem, and the anxiogenic BCs. In contrast, the BZ2 site has high affinity for the anxiolytic BZs and low affinity for the BCs, CL 218,872, and zolpidem (for structures, see Figure 1).

Since the binding of diazepam or flunitrazepam to BZ1 and BZ2 binding sites in different tissues is always stimulated by GABA, it is inferred the two BZ binding sites belong to two structurally distinct subclasses of the GABA$_A$ receptors, provisionally termed GABA$_{A1}$ and GABA$_{A2}$ (see Table 4).Recently, rat brain has been shown to contain another BZ binding site which is associated with GABA$_A$ receptors but is distinct from BZ1 or BZ2 binding sites (12, 21). The site (BZ3) is selectively labeled by PK 11195 and 4'-Cl-diazepam, both of which are virtually ineffective in displacing diazepam at BZ1 and BZ2 binding sites (12, 13, 21, Slobodyansky, this volume). The binding of PK 11195 and 4'Cl-diazepam was believed to occur

TABLE 4:   GABA$_A$ RECEPTOR SUBTYPES DEFINED BY
THE BINDING CHARACTERISTICS OF THE
ALLOSTERIC MODULATORY CENTER

GABA$_A$ receptor subtype	ALLOSTERIC MODULATORS (POSITIVE)	(NEGATIVE)	CNS AREA (RELATIVE ABUNDANCE)
GABA$_{A1}$	DIAZEPAM CLONAZEPAM ZOLPIDEM	BCCM	CEREBELLUM CORTEX
GABA$_{A2}$	DIAZEPAM	?	SPINAL CORD
GABA$_{A3}$	DIAZEPAM 4'Cl-DIAZEPAM	ISOQUINOLINE CARBOXAMIDE	OLFACTORY BULB
GABA$_{A4}$	DIAZEPAM CLONAZEPAM	BCCM	C.STRIATUM
GABA$_{A5}$	DIAZEPAM ZOLPIDEM	?	C.STRIATUM

not at GABA$_A$ receptors but rather only at a special subtype of
mitochondrial membranes which are present in central and
peripheral cells in varying abundance. However, Puia et. al.
(21) have recently demonstrated that 4'Cl-diazepam acts as a
negative allosteric modulator of GABA operated Cl$^-$ channel at
transfected GABA$_A$ receptors which are formed by the expression
of alpha$_1$, beta$_1$, and gamma$_2$ receptor subunits. The effect
is dependent on the presence of GABA and unlike that of the
anxiogenic BCs, fails to revert in the presence of flumazenil.
Preliminary evidence indicates BZ3 binding sites not only are
distributed unevenly in the brain (i.e., they are particularly
high in the olfactory bulb) but do not parallel the density of
BZ1 and BZ2 recognition site distribution as well. The data
suggests that a third GABA$_A$ receptor, GABA$_{A3}$, exists in the
brain (see Table 4).
Our binding studies with clonazepam and zolpidem in the corpus
striatum further implicate the existence of novel BZ binding
site subtypes at the allosteric center of GABA$_A$ receptors.
In the striatum, diazepam and flumazenil label the greatest
number of BZ binding sites (approx 1.6 pmol/mg prot) whereas
^{3}H-clonazepam labels only 2/3 of these binding sites (0.95
pmol/mg prot) and ^{3}H-zolpidem labels only 1/3 of these sites
(0.42 pmol/mg prot). There are two possible interpretations of

the data: A)   the c. striatum contains 3 subpopulations of BZ binding sites each representing 1/3 of the total BZ binding sites present.   The BZ1 binding sites would have high affinity for diazepam, clonazepam, and zolpidem; the BZ2 sites would have high affinity for diazepam or flumazenil only; and a last population of novel BZ sites (called BZ4) would bind diazepam, clonazepam, and beta-CCM, but not zolpidem.   B) Zolpidem and clonazepam bind to different populations of BZ binding sites, one which recognizes diazepam, clonazepam, and beta-CCM (BZ$_4$ subtype), and the other which recognizes diazepam and zolpidem (BZ$_5$ subtype).   That in the striatum the sum of clonazepam and zolpidem binding alone is close to the value observed for diazepam alone provides evidence for the existence of two different BZ binding site subtypes, one selective for clonazepam and the other selective for zolpidem.   The existence in the brain of separate BZ binding sites, one recognized by clonazepam and the other by zolpidem, is also in accordance with pharmacological observations since zolpidem elicits a strong sedative action when injected in animals (22) while clonazepam produces weak sedative effects (see Table 3).   Since binding of clonazepam and zolpidem to crude synaptic membranes of the rat striatum is enhanced by the addition of GABA and GABA$_A$ receptor agonists, it seems plausible that BZ4 and BZ5 subtypes also are included in the domain of GABA$_A$ receptors.

The structural characteristics of the different GABA$_A$ receptors listed in Table 4 remain unknown, but are likely to be different.   The GABA$_{A1}$ receptor found in cerebellum and cortex has a pharmacological behavior identical to that revealed by the GABA$_A$ receptors expressed in tumor kidney cell lines which were transfected by alpha$_1$, beta$_1$ and gamma$_2$ cDNA receptor subunits (20, 21).   Moreover, brain areas rich in GABA$_{A1}$ receptors, such as the cerebral cortex and the cerebellum (Table 4), display a high density of alpha 1 and beta 1 transcripts (17, 20, 26, 28).   The mRNA transcripts hybridize with specific oligonucleotide probes and afford the visualization of the mRNA which encodes structurally distinct GABA$_A$ receptor subunits. For the GABA$_{A2}$ receptors present in the spinal cord preliminary studies indicate levels of alpha$_1$ transcripts are lower as compared to those found in the cerebellum and cortex. Recently, a 59 kDa subunit protein was described in the spinal cord (24).   This novel subunit, like the 50 kDa alpha subunit of the GABA$_{A1}$ receptor, was photolabelled with ^{3}H-flunitrazepam which possibly indicates it is a BZ binding site.

The subtypes of GABA$_A$ receptors here identified by pharmacological differences in response to BZs, either in vivo or in vitro, awaits a precise definition of the structural distinctions among GABA$_A$ receptor subtypes.   However, recently developed technologies such as the expression of recombinant receptors via DNA transfection into cell lines which lack the receptor in question, in situ hybridization analyses for the identification of the distribution of different mRNA which encode structurally distinct GABA$_A$ receptor isoforms, and functional assays utilizing pharmacological and binding parameters in vivo and in vitro should help in elucidating this question.

REFERENCES

1. Anholt, R.R.H. (1986): *TIPS*, 12: 506-511.

2. Antkiewicz-Michaluk, L., Guidotti, A. amd Krueger, K.E. (1988): *Molecular Pharmacology*, 34: 272-278.

3. Arbilla, S., Allen, J., Wick, A. and Langer, J.Z. (1986): *Europ. J. Pharmacol.*, 130: 257-263.

4. Barnard, E.A., Burt, D.R., Darlijon, M.G., Fujita, N., Levitan, E.S., Schofield, P.R., Seeburg, P.H., Squire, M.D. and Stephenson, F.A. (1989): In: *Allosteric Modulation of Amino Acid Receptors: Therapeutic Implications*, Barnard, E. and Costa, E., eds., Raven Press, New York, pp. 19-30.

5. Bonetti, E.P., Polc, P., Laurent, J.P., Jcoc, H.P. and Haefely, W. (1987): *Neuroscience*, Suppl, 20: 582.

6. Bormann, J. and Kettenmann, H. (1988): *Proc. Natl. Acad. Sci. USA*, 80: 2072-2076.

7. Braestrup, C. and Nielsen, M. (1981): *J. Neurochem.*, 37: 333-341.

8. Braestrup, C. and Squires, R.F. (1978): *Brit. J. Psychiatry*, 133: 249-260.

9. Consalves, S.F. and Gallager, D.W. (1978): *Brain Res.*, 405: 94-99.

10. Costa, E., Alho, H., Favaron, M. and Manev, H. (1989): In: *Allosteric Modulation of Amino Acid Receptors: Therapeutic Implications*, Barnard, E. and Costa, E., eds., Raven Press, New York, pp. 3-18.

11. Farb, D.H., Borden, L.A., Chan, C.Y., Czatkowski, C.M., Gibbs, T.T. and Schiller, D.G. (1984): *Ann. N.Y. Acad. Sci.*, 435: 1-31.

12. Gee, K.W. (1987): *J. Pharmacol. Exper. Therap.*, 244: 379-383.

13. Guidotti, A., Alho, H., Berkovich, A., Cox, D.H., Ferrarese, C., Slobodyansky, E., Santi, R. and Wambebe, C. (1989): In: *Allosteric Modulation of Amino Acid Receptors: Therapeutic Implications*, Barnard, E. and Costa, E., eds., Raven Press, New York, pp. 109-123.

14. Haefely, W. (1989): In: *Allosteric Modulation of Amino Acid Receptors: Therapeutic Implications*, Barnard, E. and Costa, E., eds., Raven Press, New York, pp. 47-69.

15. Kataoka, Y., Gutman, Y., Guidotti, A. and Costa, E. (1984): *Proc. Natl. Acad. Sci. USA*, 81: 3218-3222.

16. Klepner, C.A., Lippa, A.J., Benson, D.I., Sano, M.I. and Beer, B. (1979): *Pharmacol. Biochem. Behav.*, 11: 457-462.

17. Montpied, P., Martin, B.M., Cottingham, S.L., Stubblefield, B.K., Ginns, E.I. and Paul, S.M. (1988): *J. Neurochem.*, 51: 1651-1654.

18. Olasmaa, M., Guidotti, A., Costa, E., Rothstein, J.V., Goldman, M.E., Weber, R.J. and Paul, J.M. (1989): *Lancet*, II: 491-592.

19. Overweg, J. and Binnie, C.D. (1983): In: *The Benzodiazepines, From Molecular Biology to Clinical Practice*, Costa, E.. ed., Raven Press, New York, pp. 339-347.

20. Pritchett, D.B., Sontheimer, H., Shivers, B., Ymer, S., Kattenmann, H., Schfield, P.R., and Seeburg, P.H. (1989): *Nature*, 338: 582-585.

21. Puja, G., Santi, M.R., Vicini, S., Pritchett, D.B., Seeburg, P.H. and Costa, E. (in press): *Proc. Natl. Acad. Sci. USA*.

22. Sangers, D.S. and Zivkovic, B. (1987): *Neuropharmacology*, 26: 1513-1518.

23. Santi, M.R., Cox, D.H. and Guidotti, A. (1988): *J. Neurochem.*, 50: 1080-1086.

24. Sato, T.N. and Neale, J.H. (1989): *J. Neurochem.*, Vol 52, #4: 1114-1122.

25. Schofield, P.R., Darlison, M.G., Fujita, N., Burt, D.R., Stephenson, F.A., Rodriguez, H., Rhee, L.M., Ramachandran, V.R., Glencorse, T.A., Seeburg, P.H. and Barnard, E. A. (1987): *Nature*, 328: 221-227.

26. Sequier, J.M., Richards, J.G., Malherbe, P., Price, G.W., Matwews, S. and Mohler, H. (1988): *Proc. Natl. Acad. Sci. USA*, 85: 7815-7819.

27. Thomas, J.W. and Tallman, J.F. (1983): *J. Neuroscience*, 3: 433-440.

28. Wisden, W., Morris, B.J., Darlison, M.G., Hunt, S.P. and Barnard, E.A. (1988): *Neuron*, 1: 937-947.

GABA and Benzodiazepine Receptor Subtypes,
edited by Giovanni Biggio and Erminio Costa.
Raven Press, New York © 1990.

"EX VIVO" BINDING OF ^{35}S-TBPS AS A TOOL TO STUDY THE PHARMACOLOGY OF GABA$_A$ RECEPTORS

A. Concas, E. Sanna, M. Serra, M.P. Mascia,
V. Santoro and G. Biggio

Department of Experimental Biology,
Chair of Pharmacology
University of Cagliari, ITALY

The opening of the chloride channel and the increase in the chloride permeability following the interaction of GABA with its recognition site is the most important molecular event involved in the function of central GABAergic synapses (4, 30). This mechanism previously described with electrophysiological techniques (6) can be now studied biochemically using the capability of the organophosphoric derivative t-butylbicyclophosphorothionate (TBPS) to bind to the plasma membranes (40). In fact, the binding of the radiolabelled form (^{35}S-TBPS) of this compound to high affinity recognition sites present at the level of the GABA-dependent chloride channel is very sensitive to the modulatory action exerted by most of the anxiolytic, hypnotic and anticonvulsant as well as anxiogenic, proconvulsant and convulsant drugs which specifically enhance and inhibit the function of GABAergic synapses, respectively (12, 13, 17, 32, 33, 38, 40, 41, 44).

The aim of our present work has been to verify whether the "ex vivo" binding of ^{35}S-TBPS to rat cortical membrane preparation could be a suitable tool to detect changes in the function of GABAergic transmission elicited "in vivo" by treatments which are known to alter the function of the central GABAergic synapses. Namely, we studied whether the "in vivo" increase or decrease in the availability of GABA at the synaptic level is followed by a parallel change in the binding of ^{35}S-TBPS to unwashed cortical membrane preparations from rat cerebral cortex.

The results of this study should suggest whether the enhanced or reduced function of the GABAergic synapses elicited by the different availability of GABA at the GABA$_A$ recognition site is paralleled by a conformational change of the GABA$_A$ receptor subunits which partecipate in the formation of the GABA-coupled chloride channel (3, 31, 39). If this is so, our experimental model will allow us to follow the dinamic modifications in the different molecular components involved in the structure of the GABA$_A$/benzodiazepine ionophore receptor complex. Using this experimental model we demonstrate that the "in vivo" inhibition or enhancement of GABAergic transmission results in a marked increase or decrease of ^{35}S-TBPS binding in the rat brain.

METHODOLOGICAL ASPECTS

ANIMALS: Male Sprague Dawley CD^R (Charles River, Como, Italy) weighing 180-200 g were used. They were housed, for at least one week before preparation for experiments, 6 per cage, at 24 °C with light on from 8.00 a.m. to 8.00 p.m. and had water and standard laboratory food ad libitum.

"IN VITRO" STUDIES: Benzodiazepine receptor ligands were dissolved in dimethyl sulfoxide (stock solutions 10 mM) and dilutions were made up in 50 mM Tris-Citrate buffer pH 7.4. All drugs were added to the reaction mixture at the beginning of the incubation. The control groups were incubated with an equivalent amount of solvent.

"IN VIVO" STUDIES: Benzodiazepines were given intraperitoneally 30 min before sacrifice; ß-carbolines were given intravenously 15 min before sacrifice. Isoniazid and valproic acid were administered subcutaneously and intraperitoneally, respectively, 60 min before sacrifice. Ethanol was given intragastrically 40 min before sacrifice to animals deprived of food and water 12-15 hrs before the experiment.

Benzodiazepines and ß-carbolines were dissolved in saline with one drop of Tween 80 per 5 ml. Isoniazid and valproic acid were dissolved in distilled water. Control rats received an equivalent volume of vehicle (2 ml/kg). Ethanol was diluted in a 25% solution.

FOOT-SHOCK PROCEDURE: Foot shock was provided by a stimulator which delivered a shock of 0.2 mA every 500 ms with 500 ms duration. Rats were foot shocked continuously for 5 min before sacrifice.

^{35}S-TBPS BINDING: After sacrifice the brains were rapidly removed and the cerebral cortex was dissected

out. The fresh brain tissue was homogenized with a Po-
lytron PT 10 (setting 5, for 20 s) in 50 vol of ice-
cold 50 mM Tris-citrate buffer (pH 7.4 at 25 °C) containing 100 mM NaCl, centrifuged at 20,000 x g for 20
min and reconstituted in 50 vol of Tris-citrate
buffer. ^{35}S-TBPS binding was performed as previously
described (12).

BENZODIAZEPINE RECEPTOR LIGANDS AND ^{35}S-TBPS BINDING

"IN VITRO" STUDIES: The finding that the binding of
^{35}S-TBPS is modulated in opposite manner by drugs
which facilitate or inhibit GABAergic transmission has
given a new biochemical tool to characterize the pharmacological profile of different compounds acting at
the level of the GABA$_A$ receptor complex.
Thus, the "in vitro" addition to unwashed membrane
preparations from rat cerebral cortex of GABA, GABA
mimetics and positive modulators of GABAergic transmission inhibits ^{35}S-TBPS binding. On the other hand,
GABA receptor antagonists and negative modulators of
GABAergic function elicit an opposite effect (12, 13,
17, 32, 40). In particular, benzodiazepines produce a
concentrantion-dependent inhibition of ^{35}S-TBPS binding to unwashed membrane preparation from rat cerebral cortex. However, the maximal degree of inhibition
produced by the various drugs examined is different.
In fact, we can differentiate benzodiazepines with
high efficacy which inhibit ^{35}S-TBPS binding more than
50% (Fig. 1a) from those with a lower efficacy (Fig.
1b). Among these compounds quazepam is the most effective producing a complete inhibition of ^{35}S-TBPS binding at concentration near 30 μM. On the other hand,
triazolam and alprazolam show a lower efficacy respect
to the previous drugs, an effect shared by the novel
benzodiazepine receptor ligand zolpidem, an imidazopyridine with preferential hypnotic action (23). It is
worth noting that triazolam, which has the highest affinity for benzodiazepine receptors (7), is also the
most potent benzodiazepine in decreasing ^{35}S-TBPS
binding. In fact this hypnotic produces a significant
inhibition ($-32 \pm 5.7\%$; $p < 0.01$) at the lowest concentration examined (10 nM), while higher concentrations fail to further significantly decrease ^{35}S-TBPS
binding.
In contrast to benzodiazepines, the inverse agonists
of benzodiazepine receptors (ß-carboline derivatives)
increase ^{35}S-TBPS binding in a concentration-dependent
manner (Fig. 2). However, like benzodiazepines, these
compounds show a marked difference in efficacy. Thus
DMCM is the most effective and the most potent in increasing ^{35}S-TBPS binding ($+73 \pm 14.5\%$; $p < 0.005$ at

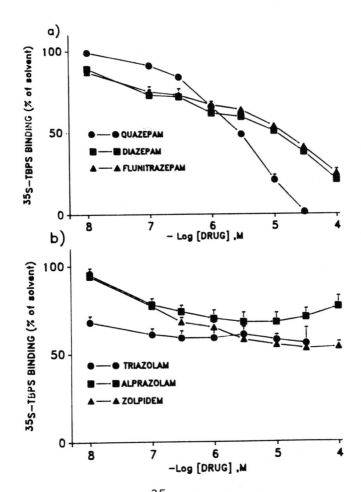

Fig. 1   INHIBITION OF ^{35}S-TBPS BINDING TO UNWASHED
RAT CORTICAL MEMBRANES BY BENZODIAZEPINE
RECEPTOR AGONISTS WITH DIFFERENT INTRINSIC
ACTIVITY.
Incubations of 2 nM ^{35}S-TBPS were maintai-
ned at 25 °C for 90 min. All points repre-
sent the means ± S.E.M. from three to six
experiments.

100 nM) while FG 7142 is the least effective enhancing
significantly ^{35}S-TBPS binding (+25 ± 4.1%; $p < 0.05$)
only at 1 μM.
All together the results suggest that by measuring
^{35}S-TBPS binding it is possible to differentiate the
benzodiazepine receptor ligands on the basis of their
efficacy in enhancing or decreasing the function of

the GABA$_A$ receptor complex. In fact, the different degree of enhancement or inhibition of ^{35}S-TBPS binding
elicited by these drugs should reflect a parallel
change in the activity of the chloride channel coupled
to GABA$_A$ receptors. Thus, these "in vitro" data strongly indicate that ^{35}S-TBPS binding might be a suitable
tool to study the function of the GABAergic synapses
"in vivo".

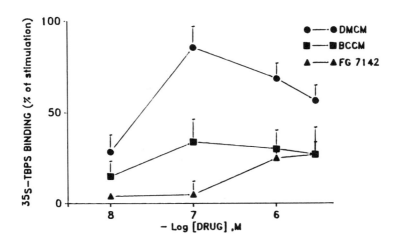

FIG. 2   ENHANCEMENT OF ^{35}S-TBPS BINDING TO UNWA-
          SHED RAT CORTICAL MEMBRANES BY BENZODIAZE-
          PINE RECEPTOR INVERSE AGONISTS.
          Incubations of 2 nM ^{35}S-TBPS were maintai-
          ned at 25 °C for 90 min. All points repre-
          sent the means ± S.E.M. from three
          experiments.

"IN VIVO" STUDIES: To verify the last conclusion, rats
were treated acutely with different benzodiazepine receptor ligands and ^{35}S-TBPS binding was measured "ex
vivo" in unwashed membrane preparations from the cerebral cortex. As expected, the intraperitoneal administration of benzodiazepines, similarly to their "in
vitro" effect, decreased ^{35}S-TBPS binding (Fig. 3).
Moreover, the intravenous administration of anxiogenic
and convulsant ß-carbolines (8, 14) produced an opposite effect.
The actions of the "in vivo" administration of positive and negative modulators of GABAergic transmission
was completely antagonized by the previous administration to rats of the specific receptor antagonist, Ro
15-1788 which per se failed to modify ^{35}S-TBPS binding
(data not shown). This finding indicates that the "in
vivo" action of these drugs are mediated by specific

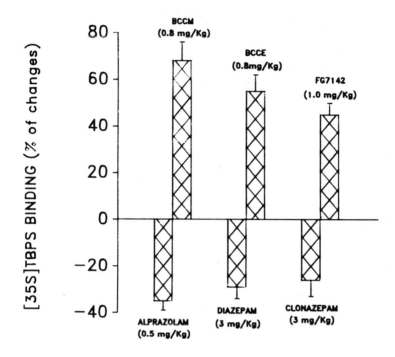

FIG. 3   OPPOSITE EFFECT OF "IN VIVO" ADMINISTRA-
TION OF BENZODIAZEPINES AND ß-CARBOLINES
ON ^{35}S-TBPS BINDING TO UNWASHED RAT CORTI-
CAL MEMBRANES.
Benzodiazepines and ß-carbolines were ad-
ministered 30 and 15 min before sacrifice,
respectively. Data are the means ± S.E.M.
from four separate experiments.

receptor interaction.
The present "in vitro" and "in vivo" data suggest that
^{35}S-TBPS binding to unwashed membrane preparations is
a sensitive index to detect the facilitatory and inhibitory actions exerted by anxiolytic and anxiogenic
drugs on the function of the $GABA_A$-dependent chloride
channel, respectively. In fact, the reduction of ^{35}S-
TBPS binding induced by GABA and benzodiazepine receptor agonists might be related to the opening state of
the ionophore. Vice versa, the increase of ^{35}S-TBPS
binding elicited by the inverse agonists and GABA antagonists should be consistent with the closing state
of the channel.

VALPROIC ACID, ISONIAZID AND ^{35}S-TBPS BINDING

To further verify this conclusion we studied wheth-

er the inhibition or the facilitation of GABAergic transmission elicited by "in vivo" administration of isoniazid or valproic acid, two drugs known to decrease and increase brain GABA content, respectively (18, 21), could be evaluated measuring "ex vivo" ^{35}S-TBPS binding in the rat cerebral cortex.
As shown in Fig. 4a a single injection of valproic a-

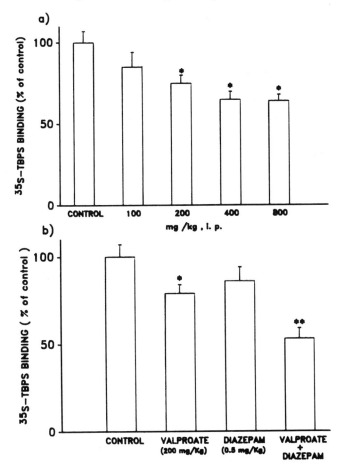

FIG. 4   "IN VIVO" ADMINISTRATION OF VALPROIC ACID DECREASES ^{35}S-TBPS BINDING TO UNWASHED RAT CORTICAL MEMBRANES: POTENTIATION BY DIAZEPAM.
a) dose curve; b) valproic acid and diazepam were administered 60 and 30 min before sacrifice, respectively. Data are the means ± S.E.M. from four separate determinations. *p < 0.05 vs control; **p < 0.05 vs valproic acid and diazepam-treated rats.

cid, produced a dose-related decrease of ^{35}S-TBPS binding in this brain area. This effect was markedly potentiated by the subsequent administration of low dose
of diazepam (0.5 mg/kg) which per se did not significantly modify ^{35}S-TBPS binding (Fig. 4b). Since valproic acid increases GABA content in the rat brain,
these results suggest that "in vivo" changes in the
availability of GABA at the synaptic level may induce
modifications in the function of the GABA-coupled
chloride channel that are detectable by measuring ^{35}S-
TBPS binding.
This hypothesis is strongly supported by the finding
that a single subcutaneous injection of isoniazid,
which reduces the availability of GABA at the receptor
site, increased ^{35}S-TBPS binding in the rat cerebral
cortex. The effect of isoniazid seems to be exclusively due to an enhancement of the maximum number of binding sites (Bmax) without a significant change in the
affinity (K_D) (Table 1). The increase of ^{35}S-TBPS bin-

TABLE 1
"IN VIVO" ADMINISTRATION OF ISONIAZID INCREASES THE
DENSITY OF ^{35}S-TBPS BINDING SITES IN THE RAT CEREBRAL
CORTEX

	^{35}S-TBPS BINDING	
	Bmax (fmol/mg prot)	K_D (nM)
Saline	1696 ± 86	72 ± 6
Isoniazid	2333 ± 142*	75 ± 9

Rats were sacrificed 60 min after isoniazid administration (300 mg/kg, s.c.). Unwashed cortical membranes were incubated in the presence of ^{35}S-TBPS (2.5 -
500 nM) at 25 °C for 90 min. Values ± S.E.M. are the
averages of five separate experiments.
*$p < 0.01$ vs saline-treated rats.

ding induced by isoniazid seems to be the consequence
of the decreased availability of GABA at the receptor
site. In fact, as shown in Fig. 5 diazepam (3 mg/kg,
i.p.), a drug that facilitate the interaction of GABA
with its recognition site (15, 19), completely antagonized the effect of isoniazid.
Taken together, these findings further indicate that
changes in ^{35}S-TBPS binding can be considered a suitable index of the functional changes of the GABAergic

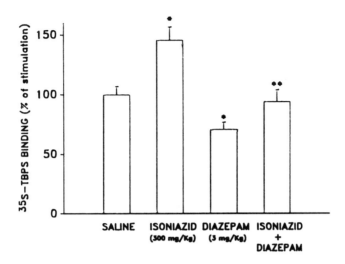

FIG. 5   "IN VIVO" ADMINISTRATION OF DIAZEPAM ANTA-
GONIZES ISONIAZID INDUCED-INCREASE OF ^{35}S-
TBPS BINDING.
Isoniazid and diazepam were administered
60 and 30 min before sacrifice, respectively. Data are the means ± S.E.M. from
three separate experiments.
*$p < 0.05$ vs saline;   **$p < 0.05$ vs
isoniazid-treated rats.

synapses. This conclusion is consistent with the data
(Fig. 3) showing that the "in vivo" administration of
negative modulators of GABAergic transmission (ß-carbolines derivatives) and the GABA receptor antagonist
bicuculline, increases ^{35}S-TBPS binding (33).
Moreover, the degeneration of specific GABAergic pathways elicited by cerebral excitotoxin injection, results in a tremendous enhancement in the density of
^{35}S-TBPS binding sites at the level of the denervated
synapses (34).

ETHANOL AND ^{35}S-TBPS BINDING

Ethanol displays pharmacological properties similar
to those of benzodiazepines and GABA mimetics (1, 24,
27, 29), and possesses both in humans and animals anxiolytic, hypnotic, sedative and myorelaxant effects
(9, 22, 25).
Accordingly different investigators have recently demonstrated that ethanol enhances "in vitro" the GABA-
stimulated ^{36}Cl$^-$ uptake into isolated cortical membrane vesicles (2, 43). This effect is similar to that of

barbiturates and opposite to those of picrotoxin and bicuculline (20, 35). These results together with previous electrophysiological (27, 29) and behavioral (26) studies suggest that the activation of $GABA_A$ -coupled chloride ionophore plays a major role in the mechanism of action of this drug.

The acute administration of ethanol (0.5-4 g/kg p.o.) elicited a dose-related inhibition of ^{35}S-TBPS binding measured "ex vivo" in unwashed membranes from rat cerebral cortex (Fig. 6). The maximal inhibitory effect of ethanol was obtained at the dose of 2 g/kg, 40 min after the administration.

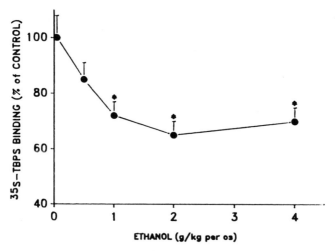

FIG. 6   "IN VIVO" ADMINISTRATION OF ETHANOL INHIBITS ^{35}S-TBPS BINDING IN THE RAT CEREBRAL CORTEX.
Ethanol was administered 40 min before sacrifice. Data are the means ± S.E.M. from four separate experiments.
*p < 0.05 vs control.

The ethanol-induced inhibition of ^{35}S-TBPS is similar to that produced by the acute intraperitoneal injection of diazepam (Fig. 3) indicating that "in vivo" administration of ethanol enhances, like benzodiazepines, the function of $GABA_A$-coupled chloride channel. However, when we compared the kinetic properties of the effect of ethanol and diazepam, Scatchard plot analysis of saturation isotherms of ^{35}S-TBPS binding indicated that, whereas diazepam (3 mg/kg) significantly reduces the density of ^{35}S-TBPS binding sites with no change in the receptor affinity, ethanol (1 g/kg) decreases the apparent affinity of ^{35}S-TBPS binding sites without modifying the Bmax value (Table 2).

TABLE 2
KINETIC CHARACTERISTICS OF ^{35}S-TBPS BINDING IN THE RAT
CEREBRAL CORTEX AFTER "IN VIVO" ADMINISTRATION OF ETHANOL AND DIAZEPAM

| | ^{35}S-TBPS BINDING | |
	Bmax (fmol/mg prot)	K_D (nM)
Control	1787 ± 47	66 ± 3
Ethanol (1 g/kg, p.o.)	1747 ± 61	87 ± 5*
Diazepam (3 mg/kg, i.p.)	1161 ± 38*	63 ± 7

Rats were sacrificed 40 and 30 min after administration of ethanol or diazepam, respectively. Unwashed cortical membranes were incubated in presence of ^{35}S-TBPS (2.5 - 500 nM) at 25 °C for 90 min. Each value represents the mean ± S.E.M. of four separate experiments. *$p < 0.05$ vs control.

Thus, the different effects on ^{35}S-TBPS binding parameters elicited by these two drugs may suggest that some of the molecular events involved in the facilitatory action of ethanol on GABA$_A$-coupled chloride channel are different from those involved in the effects of benzodiazepines.

TABLE 3
ETHANOL-INDUCED DECREASE OF ^{35}S-TBPS BINDING IN THE RAT CEREBRAL CORTEX: ANTAGONISM BY BENZODIAZEPINE RECEPTOR INVERSE AGONISTS

	^{35}S-TBPS BINDING (fmol/mg prot)	
	SOLVENT	ETHANOL (1 g/kg,p.o.)
Control	38.6 ± 1.9	27.0 ± 2.1*
ßCCE (0.6 mg/kg,i.v.)	55.9 ± 2.3*	37.0 ± 2.1
FG 7142 (12.5 mg/kg,i.p.)	54.3 ± 2.6*	39.4 ± 1.8
Ro 15-4513 (8 mg/kg,i.p.)	49.8 ± 2.2*	39.7 ± 1.5
Ro 15-1788 (8 mg/kg,i.p.)	36.3 ± 2.0	27.4 ± 2.3*

Rats were killed 60, 40, 20 and 15 min after administration of Ro 15-4513 or Ro 15-1788, ethanol, FG 7142 and ßCCE, respectively. Values are the means ± S.E.M. of four separate experiments.
*$p < 0.05$ vs. control rats.

This conclusion is supported further by the evidence that pretreatment of rats with Ro 15-1788 (8 mg/kg), while completely antagonizing diazepam-induced decrease of ^{35}S-TBPS binding (data not shown), failed to prevent the effect of ethanol (Table 3).
On the contrary, the administration of Ro 15-4513 a benzodiazepine receptor partial inverse agonist known to prevent some of the behavioral, electrophysiological and biochemical effects of ethanol (5, 28, 42), completely abolished the effect of this drug on ^{35}S-TBPS binding (Table 3). Moreover, the administration of the anxiogenic and proconvulsant ß-carboline derivatives FG 7142 (12.5 mg/kg) and ßCCE (0.6 mg/kg), like Ro 15-4513, prevented the effect of ethanol on ^{35}S-TBPS binding (Table 3).
In order to better understand the pharmacological meaning of the action of ethanol on the $GABA_A$-coupled chloride channel, we studied the effect of this compound in rats in which the GABAergic transmission was inhibited by the previous injection of isoniazid.

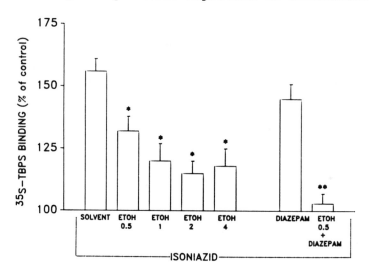

FIG. 7   DIAZEPAM ENHANCES THE ANTAGONISTIC ACTION OF ETHANOL ON ISONIAZID-INDUCED INCREASE OF ^{35}S-TBPS BINDING.
Isoniazid (300 mg/kg, s.c.), ethanol and diazepam (0.25 mg/kg, i.p.) were administered 60, 40 and 30 min before sacrifice, respectively. Data are the means ± S.E.M. from four to seven separate determinations. *p < 0.05 vs isoniazid treated rats; **p < 0.05 vs isoniazid + diazepam and isoniazid + ethanol (0.5 g/kg) treated rats.

As previously reported (Table 1) (38), the subcutaneous administration of isoniazid (300 mg/kg) elicited in 60 min a marked increase of ^{35}S-TBPS binding to cortical membrane preparations.
Moreover, ethanol administered 20 min after isoniazid almost completely reverted in a dose-dependent manner (0.5-4 g/kg) the enhancement of ^{35}S-TBPS binding elicited by this drug (Fig. 7).
The capacity of ethanol to antagonize isoniazid-induced increase of ^{35}S-TBPS binding was similar to that induced by the intraperitoneal administration of diazepam (Fig. 5). Moreover, the effect of ethanol was markedly enhanced by diazepam. In fact, the administration of a low dose of diazepam (0.25 mg/kg), which per se is uneffective on isoniazid-induced increase of ^{35}S-TBPS binding markedly potentiated the action of ethanol (0.5 g/kg) on this parameter (Fig. 7). These biochemical data indicate that "in vivo" administration of ethanol is able to antagonize the inhibitory effect of isoniazid on GABAergic synapses.
A conclusion consistent with the behavioral evidence that ethanol (1-4 g/kg) antagonizes, in a dose dependent manner, the tonic-clonic convulsions elicited by the subcutaneous administration of isoniazid (350 mg/kg) (data not shown).

STRESS AND ^{35}S-TBPS BINDING

We and others have recently demonstrated that a stressful condition modifies the function of the GABA-coupled chloride channel (10, 12, 13, 16, 36, 37, 45). Namely, our laboratory has reported that the total number of ^{35}S-TBPS binding sites is increased in the cerebral cortex of rats exposed to foot-shock stress, an effect similar to that elicited by the "in vivo" administration of anxiogenic and convulsant drugs that inhibit the GABAergic transmission (Fig. 3, Table 1; 33, 38). This finding allowed us to suggest that stress decreases the function of the GABA-dependent chloride ionophore. Accordingly, stress decreases both ^{36}Cl$^-$ efflux and uptake in a particulate membrane preparations (10, 13, 16, 37).
To further clarify the molecular mechanism involved in the inhibitory action of stress on the GABAergic transmission, more recently we studied the effect of foot-shock stress on ^{35}S-TBPS binding in the brain of rats were the GABAergic transmission was inhibited. Moreover we also analyzed the effect of stress on the seizure activity induced by isoniazid. These experiments demonstrated that foot-shock stress enhanced but not inhibited the action of isoniazid and the ß-carboline derivative FG 7142, two inhibitors of the GABAer-

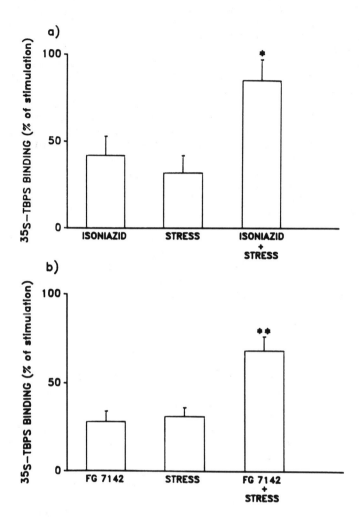

FIG. 8　FOOT-SHOCK STRESS ENHANCES THE INCREASE OF
^{35}S-TBPS BINDING INDUCED BY ISONIAZID
(PANEL a) AND FG 7142 (PANEL b) IN THE RAT
CEREBRAL CORTEX.
Foot-shock was delivered for 5 min before
sacrifice. Isoniazid (300 mg/kg, s.c.) or
FG 7142 (12.5 mg/kg i.p.) were administered 60 or 30 min before sacrifice. Data a-
re the means ± S.E.M. from six separate
determinations.
*p < 0.01 vs stress and isoniazid-treated
rats; **p < 0.05 vs stress and FG 7142-
treated rats.

gic transmission known to decrease the interaction of GABA with its recognition site (11, 21). Thus, foot-shock was delivered to rats previously treated with i-soniazid (300 mg/kg, s.c.) or with FG 7142 (12.5 mg/kg, i.p.). As previously reported (Table 1, Fig. 3; 12, 13, 38, 45) isoniazid, FG 7142 and foot-shock all increased ^{35}S-TBPS binding in the rat cerebral cortex. Moreover, as shown in Fig. 8, foot-shock markedly potentiated both the increase induced by isoniazid (+85%, $p < 0.01$, panel a) and FG 7142 (+68%; $p < 0.05$, panel b) on ^{35}S-TBPS binding.
Finally, as shown in Fig. 9 foot-shock stress also potentiated the convulsant activity of isoniazid as demonstrated by the reduced onset of seizure and the increased number of animals presenting a convulsive pattern.

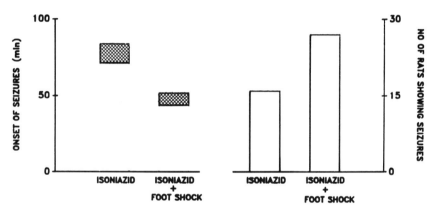

FIG. 9   FOOT-SHOCK STRESS POTENTIATES THE CONVUL-
          SANT ACTIVITY OF ISONIAZID.
          Data represent the means of six separate
          experiments. Groups of 5 rats were used
          for each experiment. The animals were ob-
          served for the apparence of convulsions
          for at least 120 min after isoniazid in-
          jection (300 mg/kg, s.c.).

The results here reported should help to clarify some of the molecular events involved in the action of foot-shock stress on the function of the GABA_A receptor complex. In fact, the biochemical and pharmacological data showing that the increase of ^{35}S-TBPS binding elicited by both isoniazid and FG 7142 together with the seizure pattern elicited by isoniazid is enhanced and not reduced by foot-shock stress indicate that foot-shock stress has an inhibitory influence on the function of the GABAergic synapses. An effect that seems specific for the GABAergic mechanism since foot-shock failed to potentiate the action of both kainic acid and stricnine (data not shown). This conclusion is supported by the finding that the effect of foot-shock stress on ^{35}S-TBPS binding was completely abolished by alprazolam (0.5 mg/kg, i.p.) and ethanol (1 g/kg, p.o.) (Fig. 10).

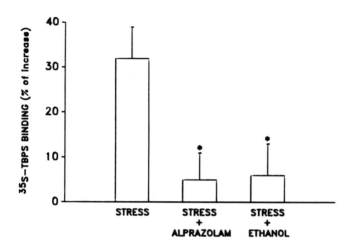

FIG. 10 ALPRAZOLAM AND ETHANOL ANTAGONIZE FOOT-SHOCK INDUCED INCREASE OF ^{35}S-TBPS BINDING IN THE RAT CEREBRAL CORTEX.
Foot-shock was delivered for 5 min before sacrifice. Alprazolam (0.5 mg/kg, i.p.) or ethanol (1 g/kg, p.o.) were administered 30 or 40 min before sacrifice. Data are the means ± S.E.M. from 4 separate experiments.
*$p < 0.05$ vs stress.

CONCLUSIONS

Our data show that the "ex vivo" measurement of ^{35}S-TBPS binding in the rat brain can be used as a suitable index to reveal an inhibition or enhancement in the function of the GABAergic transmission.
Since ^{35}S-TBPS binds to specific recognition site present on the subunits involved in the formation of the GABA-coupled chloride channel, the increase or decrease of ^{35}S-TBPS binding may reflect an opposite (negative-positive) functional state of this ion channel.
Accordingly the enhanced or reduced availability of GABA at the synaptic level plays a crucial role in the modulation of ^{35}S-TBPS binding (Fig. 4, Table 1) as

well as in the regulation of the closing and opening
state of the chloride channel (6).
This evidence might indicate that at the molecular level the changes in the binding capability of ^{35}S-TBPS
reflect the allosteric conformation of the different
subunits involved in the function of the GABA$_A$/benzo-
diazepine receptor complex.
In conclusion our data suggest that the "ex vivo" binding of ^{35}S-TBPS to the rat brain represents at present the only suitable biochemical tool to understand
the "in vivo" dinamic functional changes of the inhibitory GABAergic synapses elicited by physiological,
pharmacological and pathological conditions.

REFERENCES

1. Allan A.M. and Harris R.A., (1986): Life Sci., 39:
   2005-2015.

2. Allan A.M., Huidobro-Toro J.P., Bleck V. and Harris R.A. (1987): Alcohol, 1: 643-646.

3. Barnard E.A. and Seeburg P.H. (1988): In: Chloride
   Channels and Their Modulation by Neurotransmitters
   and Drugs, edited by G. Biggio and E. Costa, pp.
   1-18, Raven Press, New York.

4. Biggio G. and Costa E. (eds) (1988): Chloride Chan-
   nels and Their Modulation by Neurotransmitters and
   Drugs. Advances in Biochemical Psychopharmacology,
   Vol. 45, Raven Press, New York.

5. Bonetti E.P., Burkard W.P., Galb M. and Mohler H.
   (1985): Br. J. Pharmacol., 86: 463P.

6. Bormann J., Hamill O.P. and Sakmann B.J. (1987):
   J. Physiol., 385: 243-286.

7. Braestrup C. and Nielsen M. (1986): In: Benzodia-
   zepine/GABA receptors and Chloride Channels:
   Structural and Functional Properties, edited by
   R.W. Olsen and J.C. Venter, pp. 167-184, Alan R.
   Liss, New York.

8. Braestrup C., Schmiechen R., Neef G., Nielsen M.
   and Petersen E.N. (1982): Science, 216: 1241-1243.

9. Cole J.O. and Davis J.M. (1975) In: American Handbook of Psychiatry, edited by D.X. Freedman and
   J.E. Dyrud, pp. 427-440, Basic Books, New York.

10. Concas A., Mele S. and Biggio G. (1987): Eur. J.

Pharmacol., 135: 423-427.

11. Concas A., Salis M., Serra M., Corda M.G. and Biggio G. (1983): Eur. J. Pharmacol., 89: 179-181.

12. Concas A., Serra M., Atsoggiu T. and Biggio G. (1988): J. Neurochem., 51: 1868-1876.

13. Concas A., Serra M., Corda M.G. and Biggio G. (1988) In: Chloride Channels and their Modulation by Neurotransmitters and Drugs, edited by G. Biggio and E. Costa, pp. 227-246, Raven Press, New York.

14. Corda M.G., Blaker W.D., Mendelson W.B., Guidotti A. and Costa E. (1983): Proc. Natl. Acad. Sci. U.S.A., 80: 2072-2076.

15. Costa E. and Guidotti A. (1979): Ann. Rev. Pharmacol. Toxicol., 19: 531-545.

16. Drugan R.C., Morrow A.L., Weizman R., Weizman A., Deutsch S.I., Crawley J.N. and Paul S.M. (1989): Brain Res., 487: 45-51.

17. Gee K.W., Lawrence L.J. and Yamamura H.I. (1986): Mol. Pharmacol., 30: 218-225.

18. Godyn Y., Heiner L., Mark J. and Mandel P. (1969): J. Neurochem., 16: 869-873.

19. Haefely W., Kyburz E., Gerecke M. and Mohler H. (1985): In: Advances in Drug Research, pp. 165-322, Academic Press, London.

20. Harris R.A. and Allan A.M. (1985): Science, 228: 1108-1110.

21. Horton R.W. (1980): Brain Res. Bull., 5: 605-608.

22. Koob G.F., Strecker R.E. and Bloom F. (1980): Subst. Alcohol Actions Misuse, 1: 447-457.

23. Langer S.Z., Depoortere H., Sanger D., George P., Zivkovic B., Arbilla S., Lloyd K.G. and Bartholini G. (1985): J. Neurochem., 44: 179-187.

24. Liljequist S. and Engel J.A. (1982): Psychopharmacology, 78: 71-75.

25. Liljequist S. and Engel J.A. (1984): Pharmacol. Biochem. Behav., 18: 521-525.

26. Mendelson W.B., Martin J.V., Wagner R., Roseberry C., Skolnick P., Weissman B.A. and Squires R. (1985): Eur. J. Pharmacol., 108: 63-70.

27. Mereu G. and Gessa G.L. (1985): Brain Res., 360: 325-330.

28. Mereu G., Passino N., Carcangiu P., Boi V. and Gessa G.L. (1987): Eur. J. Pharmacol., 135: 453-454.

29. Nestoros J.N. (1980): Science, 209: 708-710.

30. Olsen R.W. and Venter J.C. (1986): In: Benzodiazepine/GABA Receptors and Chloride Channels, Structural and Functional Properties: Receptor Biochemistry and Methodology, Vol. 5, Alan R. Liss, New York.

31. Pritchett D.B., Luddens H. and Seeburg P.H. (1989): Science, 245: 1389-1392.

32. Ramanjaneyulu R. and Ticku M.K. (1984): J. Neurochem., 42: 221-229.

33. Sanna E., Concas A., Serra M. and Biggio G. (1989): Eur. J. Neurosci., Suppl. 2: 287.

34. Sanna E., Serra M., Pepitoni S. and Biggio G. (1989): Brain Res., 501: 144-149.

35. Schwartz R.D., Skolnick P., Seale T.W. and Paul S.M. (1986): In: GABAergic Transmission and Anxiety, edited by G. Biggio and E. Costa, pp. 33-49, Raven Press, New York.

36. Schwartz R.D., Wess M.J., Labarca R., Skolnick P. and Paul S.M. (1987): Brain Res., 411: 151-155.

37. Serra M., Concas A., Atsoggiu T. and Biggio G. (1989): Neurosci. Research Comm., 4: 41-50.

38. Serra M., Sanna E. and Biggio G. (1989): Eur. J. Pharmacol., 164: 385-388.

39. Shivers B.D., Killisch I., Sprengel R., Sontheimer H., Kohler M., Schofield P.R. and Seeburg P.H. (1989): Neuron., 3: 327-337.

40. Squires R.F., Casida J.E., Richardson M. and Saederup E. (1983): Mol. Pharmacol., 23: 326-336.

41. Supavilai P. and Karobath M. (1984): J. Neurosci., 4: 1193-1200.

42. Suzdak P.D., Glowa J.R., Crawley J.N., Schwartz R.D., Skolnick P. and Paul S.M. (1986): Science, 234: 1243.

43. Suzdak P.D., Schwartz R.D., Skolnick P. and Paul S.M. (1986): Proc. Natl. Acad. Sci. USA, 83: 4071-4075.

44. Trifiletti R.R., Snowman A.M. and Snyder S.H. (1984): Mol. Pharmacol., 26: 470-476.

45. Trullas R., Havoundjian H. and Skolnick P. (1987): J. Neurochem., 49: 968-974.

GABA and Benzodiazepine Receptor Subtypes,
edited by Giovanni Biggio and Erminio Costa.
Raven Press, New York © 1990.

DIFFERENTIAL ACTION OF VARIOUS ALLOSTERIC MODULATORS
OF $GABA_A$ RECEPTOR UPON THE SPONTANEOUS
DISCHARGE RATE OF NIGRAL NEURONS "IN VIVO"

Giampaolo Mereu and Giovanni Biggio

Department of Experimental Biology, "Bernardo Loddo"
Section of Neuroscience
University of Cagliari, 09100 Cagliari, Italy

Substantia nigra (SN) is a key area for the γ-aminobutiric acid (GABA) mediated pre- and post-synaptic input to basal ganglia. Its well known cytoarchitecture (see ref. 10 for review) separates the dorsal portion of SN, the pars compacta (PC), which contains dopamine (DA) cells, from the ventral portion, the pars reticulata (PR) where, GABAergic striato-nigral terminals and GABAergic cells are located. GABA activity is very prominent in PR. Indeed, PR cells contain the highest concentration of GABA and glutamic acid decarboxylase of any other mammalian brain area (1,32) which appear coupled to an abundant presence of benzodiazepine (BDZ) receptors (33).

In the nervous system, binding studies have revealed an area specific heterogeneity for the affinity of different BDZ ligands (17,36,38). On this basis, the high affinity BDZ recognition sites have been distinguished into three subtypes called BDZ 1, BDZ 2, and the peripheral type BDZ 3. They have been found in the brain of most mammals, human included (4,8). However, recent studies suggest that such a classification is probably too general since the prototypic GABA/BDZ complex actually appears a heteropolymeric structural protein composed of five subunits (2 α + 2 β + 1 γ or δ), or their multiple variants, each showing different affinity and different electro-physiological responsiveness to GABA and BDZ ligands (2) as well as a different regional distribution (33,37). Although the relationship between the pharmacologically defined BDZ receptor subtypes and subunit variants of $GABA_A$ receptor is only now being clarified (30, 31), it is worth noting that the previously described BDZ 1 and BDZ 2 receptors are abundant but differen-tially localized in the rat PR: the former on soma and dendrites of intrinsic neurons, the latter on axons or terminals of the striato-nigral pathway (7,18). Moreover, immunocytochemical studies have shown that in the SN-PR the α-subunits of GABA receptors are largely present in both axonal terminal and perikarya (40), while the hybridization signal for the β-subunits is much weaker (37).

Coherently with this neuronal organization of GABAergic nature, PR cells have proven to be extremely sensitive to the action of various positive (anxiolytics, sedatives, hypnotics, anticonvulsants, anesthetics, etc.) as well as negative (anxiogenics, analeptics, pro-convulsants, etc.) modulators of GABAergic transmission. Indeed, through an allosteric inter-action with specific recognition sites of the GABA/BDZ/Cl$^-$ ionophore supramolecular complex (9), positive modulators increase, while negative ones decrease, GABA-mediated Cl$^-$ conductance (2,19,29,31,42). Therefore, positive modulators depress while negative modulators stimulate the spontaneous high rate firing of PR neurons (14,22,23,25,34,43,44).

From the functional point of view, PR neurons appear to be greatly involved in motor coordination since they comprise a population of short-axon cells which interface between various convergent afferents (mainly from caudate-putamen, globus pallidus, and nucleus accumbens) and the DAergic cells of the pars compacta. Moreover, the long-axon PR cells project to several movement-related areas, including the superior colliculus, thalamus, striatum, and reticular formation (see 1,10,11,25 for references and review). Furthemore,because of the tonic inhibitory (GABAergic) control exerted by PR neurons upon DAergic cells and their 20 times higher sensitivity to GABA, depression of PR cells firing by the systemic administration of GABA agonists and ethanol (ETH) results in a parallel activation of DAergic cells (14,25,26,44). This mechanism might be relevant in considering that DAergic cells have shown, among other features, to constitute the biological substrate for the euphoria and artificial reward by ETH and other drugs of abuse (25,26). Another point of interest would be to associate the high sensitivity of PR cells to GABAergic agents with the crucial role played by these cells in the control of seizure propagation, GABA-mediated ETH withdrawal seizures, and the GABA-mediated activity of anticonvulsant drugs (11,13,41,45).

For all mentioned above, PR neurons are in the focus of growing interest for neuropharmacologists and neurophysiologists. In the following pages we will attempt to present an overview of the recent studies on the response of these neurons to the action of various modulators of GABA receptors "in vivo."

EXPERIMENTAL MODEL

Data herein reported were obtained by monitoring extracellular action potentials from single cells of PR in adult rats. Details on the electrophysiological methodology, cell identification, and animal preparation have already been published (20-26). Since PR cells are sensitive to anesthetics (see section 8), several experiments had to be performed in awake and locally anesthetized animals. In these cases, the instructions of NIH issue "Guide for Care and Use of Laboratory Animals" were carefully followed.

1. AGONISTS OF BDZ RECEPTORS

BDZs are considered "positive" modulators of $GABA_A$ receptor function in that they enhance Cl^- channels opening frequency (19,42), thereby hyperpolarizing the cellular membrane and reducing the spontaneous firing. In line with this evidence, we and others have found that PR cells are extremely sensitive to i.v. injection of several BDZs such as flurazepam (FLUR), diazepam (DIAZ), alprazolam (ALPRAZ), triazolam (TRIAZ), flunitrazepam (FLUN), and quazepam (QUAZ) (21,22,34,43). On the basis of the dosage effective in inhibiting basal rate by 50% (ED_{50}), the rank order of potency of these six representatives of the BDZ class was FLUN >> TRIAZ >> ALPRAZ > DIAZ > FLUR >> QUAZ (see Table 1) which correlates well with their known sedative efficacy in humans. However, the pattern of the

TABLE 1:
ED_{50} OF VARIOUS POSITIVE AND NEGATIVE MODULATORS OF BZD RECEPTOR ON PR ACTIVITY

DRUG	ED_{50}	S.E.	No. of cells
POSITIVE			
Quazepam	>10,000	520	8
Flurazepam	2,500	125	12
Alpidem	1,620	150	10
Diazepam	542	23	36
Alprazolam	490	42	6
Triazolam	156	38	8
ZK 93423	134	36	20
Zolpidem	79	28	28
Flunitrazepam	21.3	0.8	18
NEGATIVE			
FG 7142	>> 25,000	1,000	12
Ro 5-4864	4,220	320	6
Ro 15-4513	490	36	22
β-CCE	232	24	18
DMCM	143	12	15
β-CCM	95	8	18

Table 1: The ED_{50} (effective dose 50) is the dose producing the 50% of firing rate change with respect to baseline. Each value is the mean ± S.E. obtained from the reported number of cells. Dosages (μg/Kg i.v.) refer to single bolus injection.

inhibitory effect was different within these drugs (Fig. 1). Thus, while QUAZ (10.0 mg/kg), FLUR (8.0 mg/kg), and DIAZ (5.0 mg/kg) produced supramaximal and long-lasting depression of the firing rate ranging between 40% and 60% of baseline, in the majority (82%) of tested cells FLUN (0.2 mg/kg) completely, but temporarily, abolished the electrical activity. TRIAZ was highly efficacious and the most persistent ligand we tested since 1.0 mg/kg of this drug silenced PR cells for up to 2-3 hours.

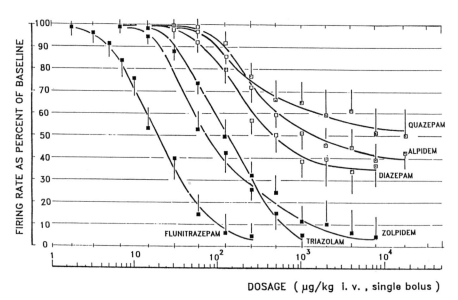

DOSAGE (μg/kg i. v. , single bolus)

Fig. 1: Dose-response plot of the inhibitory effects elicited by various positive BDZ ligands on the spontaneous discharge rate of PR neurons. Drugs were injected i.v. into a previously cannulated femoral vein. Each point (± S.E.M.) was obtained by averaging the response of 6-36 neurons. Experimental protocol followed single bolus regimen; thus, only one dose and one cell per rat was studied.

2. INVERSE AGONISTS OF BDZ RECEPTORS

We were first in demonstrating that different anxiogenic, proconvulsant, and convulsant β-carboline (β-CB) derivatives were able not only to antagonize BDZ-induced inhibition of PR cells but also to activate, per se, the cell firing up to 120-140% above basal rates (22,24). As shown in Fig. 2, the rank order of potency of these drugs was β-CCM > DMCM > β-CCE >> FG 7142. It has been argued that this effect, among others, is due to the "negative" modulatory action exerted by β-CBs upon the GABA_A/BDZ receptor. This action would trigger a reduced interaction between GABA and its recognition site, thereby decreasing the opening frequency of the GABA-gated Cl⁻ channels without changing their single conductance or opening duration (29,42). Accordingly, β-CBs can induce a spectrum of actions exactly opposite of that of BDZs themselves. For this reason β-CBs are defined "inverse agonists" of BDZ receptors (see: 4 for refs.). Moreover, since all β-CB effects, including stimulation of PR firing, are readily abolished by specific BDZ receptor antagonists (see below), it supports the idea that β-CBs might interact with the same recognition site of BDZs.

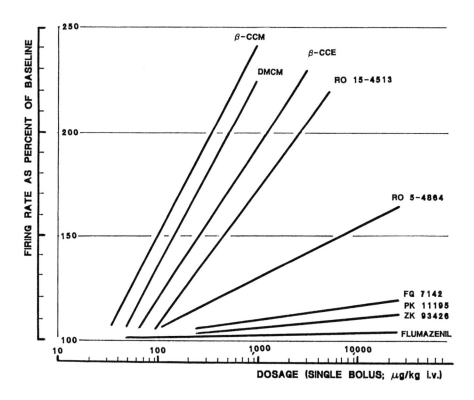

Fig. 2 : Regression lines showing the dose-related effect of various negative agonists and antagonists of BDZ receptors on the firing of SN-PR neurons. Each point represents the mean change of activity at the peak effect averaged for the number of cells tested (N=6-14). To avoid residual effects, only one dose and one cell per rat was studied.

3. ANTAGONISTS OF BDZ RECEPTORS

The best known "pure" antagonist of BDZ receptors is flumazenil (FLUM or Ro 15-1788) (15). In several paradigms, including the firing rate of PR cells, this drug appears completely devoid of intrinsic effects even at very high doses (10.0 mg/kg). Nevertheless doses as low as 0.2 mg/kg are usually fully sufficient to revert and prevent both depression and excitation induced by BDZs and β-CBs, respectively, upon the spontaneous electrical activity of PR neurons (22,34). By computerized analysis of the firing pattern of these cells we observed also that the increase in the interspike interval and the reduction of burst production, triggered by several BDZ positive modulators, was reconstituted to exactly pre-drug values by FLUM (see Fig. 3). In a similar fashion, the opposite changes of these parameters elicited by negative modulators were also eliminated by FLUM (not shown).

Other compounds have been proposed as BDZ antagonists (15,16). One of these, Ro 15-4513, has stimulated great interest because of its claimed inertness yet associated to rather selective antagonistic properties against not only BDZs but also versus ETH (39). Further tests have then revealed that Ro 15-4513 behaves, similarly to β-CBs, as a BDZ-inverse agonist (20). As shown in Fig. 2, Ro 15-4513 produced,in our study, a marked activation of PR cells which was blocked by low doses (0.5 - 1.0 mg/kg) of FLUM (20). We have also examined the β-CB derivative ZK 93426. Like FLUM, ZK 93426 was without effect up to 10.0 mg/kg, yet it completely antagonized the firing rate changes of different positive and negative BDZ receptor modulators in a range of doses of 0.5-2.0 mg/kg (23). Isoquinoline carboxamide PK 11195, an antagonist of peripheral BDZ 3 receptors, was found slightly excitatory (less than 10%) when injected at high dosage (> 8.0 mg/kg). Nevertheless, 2.0 mg/kg of PK 11195 antagonized the stimulant response induced on PR cells by the BDZ derivative 4'-chlorodiazepam (Ro 5-4864; 2.0-4.0 mg/kg), a selective ligand for the BDZ 3 receptors, but failed to interfere with the action of both positive and negative ligands for the central type of BDZ receptors (21).

4. NON BDZ AGONISTS OF BDZ RECEPTORS

ZK 93423 is a β-CB derivative; however it possesses BDZ-like effects. In line with this property, we found that the i.v. injection of 0.1-1.0 mg/kg of ZK 93423 produced a profound depression of the firing of PR cells up to complete cessation of their activity (23). This effect was reversed by DMCM and potentiated by DIAZ. Moreover, the rate inhibition by ZK 93423 was abolished and prevented by BDZ antagonists such as ZK 93426 and FLUM. The latter compound, however, was found to be much less potent against ZK 93423 than versus DIAZ.

Recent advances in the knowledge of the molecular biology of the GABA/BDZ receptor complex are compatible with the view that drugs acting with different potencies and efficacies at a given

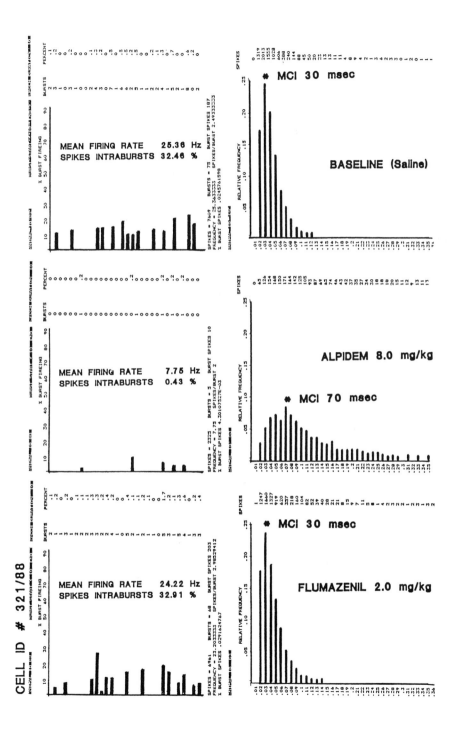

Fig. 3:   Computerized   analysis   of   discharge   pattern   of   PR
           neurons.   Distribution   of   inter-spike   intervals   (right
           panels)   and   percent   of   burst   production,   i.e.,   percent
           of   spikes   occuring   within   bursts,   (left   panels)   are
           shown.   Extracellular   action   potentials   were   sampled
           for   5   min,   starting   3   min   after   termination   of   i.v.
           administration   of   saline   (baseline),   alpidem,   and   fluma-
           zenil.   Note   that   the   reduction   of   burst   activity   and
           the   lengthiness   of   the   most   common   inter-spike   interval
           (MCI)   induced   by   alpidem   were   brought   back   to   almost
           exactly   baseline   values   by   flumazenil.   Analogous
           results   were   obtained   with   all   other   BZD   ligands
           studied.

-----

subtype   of   BDZ   receptors   may   induce   more   selective   pharmacological   effects   than   those   ligands   which   do   not   discriminate   among
receptor   subtypes.   For   this   purpose   zolpidem   and   alpidem,   two
imidazopyridines   with   high   affinity   for   the   BDZ   recognition
sites   of   subtype   1,   have   recently   been   selected   (17,38).   Indeed,
the   therapeutical   interest   of   these   novel   ligands   rests   on   the
fact   that,   while   zolpidem   (ZOLP)   has   been   presented   as   a
hypnotic,   alpidem   (ALP)   appears   to   be   a   preferential   anxiolytic
(17).   Overall   both   of   them   seem   to   lack   other   typical   actions
and   side   effects   of   BDZs,   such   as   myorelaxation,   ataxia,
synergism   with   ETH,   residual   effect,   tolerance,   and   amnesia
(35).   When   compared   to   DIAZ   in   our   experimental   paradigm,   ZOLP
and   ALP   produced   a   dose-dependent   (0.03 - 8.0 mg/kg i.v. as
single   bolus)   inhibition   of   the   firing   of   SN-PR   cells.   However,
as   shown   in   Table   1,   ZOLP   was   found   to   be   more   potent   than   DIAZ
and   ALP   (their ED_{50} were   79 ± 23;   542 ± 23   and   1,620 ± 125
μg/Kg,   respectively),   and   much   more   efficacious.   When   a
supramaximal   dose   (4.0 mg/kg)   of   ZOLP   was   injected   in   a   single
bolus,   it   completely   silenced   all   cells   tested   (8/8)   whereas   the
same   dose   of   either   DIAZ   or   ALP   produced,   in   6/6   cells,   a
typical   maximal   inhibition   of   about   55%   with   respect   to   baseline
(Fig. 4).
    The   effect   of   these   three   drugs   was   also   tested   by
administering   exponentially   increasing   (ratio   2)   cumulative
doses   starting   at   0.015   mg/kg.   Clear   signs   of   rapid   tolerance
(tachyphylaxis)   were   observed,   especially   for   DIAZ   and   ZOLP.
Table   2   shows   that   when   supramaximal   cumulative   doses   of   ZOLP,
ALP,   and   DIAZ   were   reached,   they   produced   an   inhibition   of
firing   reduced   by   22.40,   3.47   and   14.5%   respectively,   when
compared   to   the   same   dose   injected   as   a   single   bolus.
    To   determine   whether   the   firing   inhibition   produced   by   the
two   imidazopyridines   were   actually   mediated,   like   that   of   DIAZ,
through   the   activation   of   central   BDZ   receptors,   a   low   dose   (0.5
mg/kg)   of   FLUM   (Ro   15-1788)   was   administered   5   to   20   min   after
the   drugs .   As   expected   for   DIAZ,   a   single   injection   (0.5 mg/kg)
of   FLUM   was   able   to   completely   cancel   the   effect   of   ZOLP,   ALP,
and   DIAZ,   bringing   the   discharge   rate   and   firing   pattern   back   to

the basal values (see Figs. 3 & 4). Moreover, pretreatment with FLUM (0.5 - 2.0 mg/kg) completely prevented the drugs-induced inhibition (not shown).

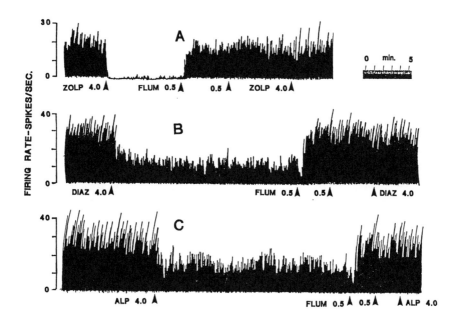

Fig. 4: Integrated rate histograms showing the inhibitory effect of an i.v. overdose (4.0 mg/kg) of zolpidem (ZOLP), A, diazepam (DIAZ), B, and alpidem (ALP), C. As a rule, while maximal inhibition produced by DIAZ and ALP was in a range of 50 to 60% with respect to basal rates, the same dose of ZOLP completely silenced cells activity. Thereafter, 0.5 mg/kg of flumazenil (FLUM) restored basal rate and prevented the effect of subsequent administration of the agonist. No further changes were induced by higher doses of flumazenil.

MAXIMAL INHIBITION OF SNR CELLS' ACTIVITY ELICITED BY
DIAZEPAM, ALPIDEM AND ZOLPIDEM (4.0 mg/kg i.v.)

DRUG	SINGLE BOLUS	CUMULATIVE DOSE	Δ-PERCENT OF SINGLE BOLUS	P (Δ) <
	% OF INHIBITION			
Diazepam	64.32 $\pm$ 4.31	55.22 $\pm$ 3.24	14.15	0.05
Alpidem	60.82 $\pm$ 3.82	58.71 $\pm$ 2.72	3.47	N.S.
Zolpidem	94.24 $\pm$ 8.31	73.13 $\pm$ 4.22	22.40	0.01

Table 2: Drug response were evaluated at the peak effect (2-5 min after injection) as percent change of the firing rate with respect to baseline. Each value is the mean $\pm$ S.E.M. of 9 to 18 cells. Statistic of difference was estimated by the Student's t test. Cumulative dose was reached by administering the drug in exponentially increasing doses starting from 15 μg/kg. In 3 experiments initial dosage of zolpidem was 7.5 μg/kg.

5. PROLONGED EXPOSURE OF PR CELLS TO BDZ LIGANDS

Prolonged exposure to BDZs has been shown to alter several types of response to either BDZ agonists, antagonists or inverse agonists of BDZ receptors (see 47). In particular, after sub-chronic (2 to 4 weeks) treatment with BDZ agonists, PR cells appear less responsive to a challenge of systemic DIAZ but more excitable by DMCM (47). They also show a reduced ability of FLUR to potentiate the inhibitory response of iontophoretically applied GABA. Furthermore, after subchronic DIAZ, FLUM was found both to produce pro-convulsant effect and to activate basal firing of PR neurons, two actions characteristically induced by BDZ-inverse agonists in normal animals. Hence, the FLUM response has been considered a correlate of withdrawal syndrome induced by prolonged treatment with BDZ agonists (47). It has, however, been observed that the above results were obtained when DIAZ was still present in rats which were also under chloral hydrate anesthesia during the experimental procedure. To overcome these problems, and to investigate the ability of other BDZ receptor ligands to induce electrophysiological signs of dependence, we have recently repeated the experiment in awake, locally anesthetized rats. For two weeks animals received three daily subcutaneous injections (3x3.0 mg/kg) of either DIAZ or ZOLP (see section 4). Twenty-four and seventy-two hours from the final injection basal activity of PR cells was sampled before administering increasing doses (0.5+0.5+1.0+2.0 mg/kg) of FLUM i.v. The results summarized in Fig. 5 show that the sub-chronic treatment with DIAZ produces a slight (but not statistically significant) depression of spontaneous discharge rate of cells which was, however, activated above control levels by FLUM. On the contrary, a similar pre-treatment with ZOLP failed to modify both spontaneous activity and the null response to FLUM. These different responses to FLUM cannot be explained by a weaker activity of ZOLP upon PR cells since the drug appears much more potent and efficaceous than DIAZ in inhibiting the spontaneous firing of these neurons (see section 4).

It is concluded that, by using the paradigm of SN-PR firing response, ZOLP is less capable of producing electrophysiological signs of dependence and, presumably, tolerance (Mereu, preliminary data). These results are in agreement with other clinical and behavioral studies (35), and further point out the peculiar pharmacological profile of ZOLP as BDZ receptor ligand.

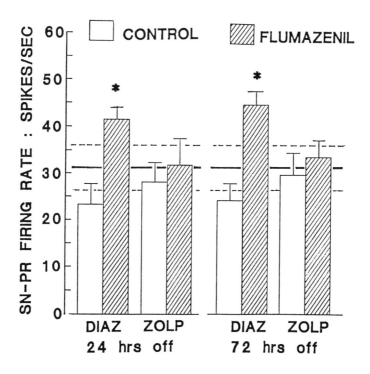

Fig. 5: Effect of sub-chronic (14 days) treatment with DIAZ and ZOLP on the spontaneous firing rate of PR neurons (open bars) and on the response to FLUM (hatched bars). Horizontal stippled band indicates the mean ($\pm$ S.E.M.) basal rate of these cells in normal or saline treated animals which is not modified by FLUM. See text for drug regimen. * $P < 0.05$ versus control values.

Conversely to BZDs, repeated treatment with central stimulants have been reported to produce sensitization to the drug or "chemical kindling". Accordingly, in our laboratory it has recently been found (5,6) that chronic treatment with the β-carbolines βCCE or FG 7142 lead to a long lasting reduction of the threshold for the convulsant or proconvulsant effects induced by βCCE, DMCM, and Ro 15-4513, as well as a decrease in density of low affinity GABA receptors, an attenuation of the anticonvulsant efficacy of DIAZ, and a reduction of GABA-stimulated $^{36}Cl^-$ uptake. In view of the involvement of PR neurons in the genesis and control of generalized seizure, we studied their basal activity and their responsiveness to FG 7142, DMCM and DIAZ in rats treated for 15 days with 2x25.0 mg/kg of FG 7142. Surprisingly, no differences in the sensitivity of the above BDZ ligands were found. However, in the rats treated with FG 7142, the frequency distribution of basal firing rate/cells showed an increase in the number of those cells firing at highest rates (21).

6. BARBITURATES

Like BDZs, barbiturates have been shown to enhance GABA receptor response (19) as well as binding of GABA to GABA receptors (27). At variance of BDZs (42), biophysical analysis of the GABA-gated chloride ion channels have, however, revealed that pentobarbital (PBARB) decreases the frequency of Cl^- channel opening, yet increasing the average open channel lifetime and prolonging the duration of the opening channel burst evoked by GABA (19). As a net result, PBARB potentiates membrane hyperpolarization and firing inhibition mediated by GABA. Accordingly, i.v. administration of barbiturates, such as the anesthetic-hypnotic PBARB (0.3-80 mg/kg), and the anticonvulsant phenobarbital (5-50 mg/kg), reduces or suppresses the firing of PR neurons dose dependently (20,21,45). Moreover, this effect can be antagonized by GABA antagonists, such as bicuciline and picrotoxin (14,45), and also by inverse agonists of BDZ receptors, such as DMCM and Ro 15-4513, but not by BDZ receptor antagonists such as FLUM (20,21).

7. ETHANOL

Alhough the molecular mechanism through which ETH interferes with CNS functions has not completely clarified, a body of evidence supports that ETH facilitates the Cl^- channel opening (see 20 for refs.), thereby "mimicking", or at least potentiating, the synaptic action of GABA.

In line with this evidence, we have found (25) that systemic administration of clinically relevant doses of ETH (0.2 - 2.0 g/kg) produces a marked inhibitory effect on the firing of PR cells (24). The effect was reversed by picrotoxin and bicuciline, as well as by different β-CBs and Ro 15-4513. Conversely, the ETH induced depression of PR neurons was potentiated by muscimol, a GABA receptor agonist, and by DIAZ. FLUM removed the potentiating effect of DIAZ but failed to modify, per se, the depression of firing rate produced by ETH. Moreover, the delivery of ETH by micropressure directly onto the somata of PR neurons produced a slowing of their firing, sensitivity to the drug being about 3 fold higher than that showed by SN-DAergic cells (26). Such inhibition was prevented by concurrent ejection of bicuculline onto the cell (25). These results provide a further, even indirect, support to the hypothesis that ETH would inhibit the firing of PR neurons via a GABA-like mechanism (25,26).

8. OTHER CNS DEPRESSANTS
    Besides ETH, BDZs and barbiturates, other drugs known to enhance GABAergic transmission, such as muscimol (0.2 - 4.0 mg/kg), valproic acid (5-500 mg/kg), chloral hydrate (50-400 mg/kg), urethan (100-600 mg/kg), and halothane (0.3 - 4.0%), reduce the firing of PR cells dose dependently (12,25,28). This finding might be relevant in considering that some of the above drugs (e.g., chloral hydrate) are currently used as general anesthetics for electrophysiological single cell studies "in vivo". Infact we observed that the use of such preparations may mask a number of physiological and pharmacological responses of PR cells and also of neighboring DA cells of SN-PC (12,14,44,45). Moreover, firing inhibition of PR neurons appears to be an effect restricted to GABA mimetic depressants only. In fact, other non-GABAergic anesthetics, such as ketamine and nitrous oxide, or anticonvulsants such as phenytoin, ethosuximide, and carbamazepine do not alter or even accelerate, in certain cases (e.g. nitrous oxide, ketamine, and ethosuximide) the basal firing rate of these neurons (21,28,45).

9. MUTUAL INTERACTION BETWEEN PC AND PR CELLS
    Several studies have described the control exerted by nigral PR cells upon DA cells of PC (14,44). Thus, inhibition of PR cells by the systemic administration of GABAergic drugs, ETH, and certain anesthetics usually results in a biphasic response of DAergic cell activity. Low doses of these agents activate DA cells through a disinhibitory process (25,26), while high doses can directly affect DA cells leading to their firing inhibition (25). Such a mechanism, however, does not appear to be bidirectional since activation of PR firing by GABAergic antagonists does not inhibit DA cells, but rather excites them (10,14,21,44).
    Vice versa, DA cells might also control PR cells. Indeed, endogenous DA, released by DAergic dendrites of PC neurons innervating PR, appears to modulate the GABA tone of striatal afferents to PR cells (46).

DISCUSSION

    The elevated sensitivity shown by PR cells to various positive and negative modulators of GABAergic transmission emphasizes the feasibility of their spontaneous firing as a high resolution "in vivo" paradigm. Regarding those allosteric modulators of GABA receptors binding to the BDZ recognition sites, a number of novel and interesting ligands are now available. However, the intrinsic effect of these drugs upon PR cells does not appear to be necessarily linked to the chemical class they belong to. Accordingly, on the basis of their effect on the spontaneous firing of PR cells, various BDZ receptor ligands may be classified into three categories: agonists, inverse agonists, and antagonists. It is relevant that the direction of action and potency manifested by these compounds in our paradigm are usually well correlated with their biochemical and behavioral effects both in animal and human. For instance, the most potent and efficacious inhibitors of PR firing are fast hypnotics in the clinical use. Indeed the BDZ receptor ligands TRIAZ, FLUN, and ZOLP, as well as the hypnotic anesthetics PBARB, and chloral hydrate, can completely stop the activity of PR cells. On the other hand, BDZ receptor ligands with pharmacological profile of anxiolytic and/or anticonvulsants have a relatively mild action, reducing firing up to 40-50% of basal rate. In this category we might include DIAZ, ALP, FLUR and QUAZ.

The reason for such differentiation is not clear. It might depend on the pharmacokinetic properties of each drug, degree of affinity for the BDZ receptors, intrinsic activity, and preferential interaction for one of BDZ receptor subtypes, or a combination of two or more of these factors. Regarding the heterogenous distribution of the α subunit of GABA_A receptors, which contains the recognition site for BDZs (2), it is worth noting that they are abundant in the PR (37). Whatever the rationale for these differentiated actions, there is no doubt that the effects exerted by either positive or negative BDZ ligands upon PR cells are due to their specific interaction with the BDZ recognition site(s) because the effects are rapidly cancelled by low doses of the selective BDZ antagonist FLUM.

Since many positive modulators of GABA_A receptors have anticonvulsant properties, while the negative ones have convulsant or proconvulsant activities, it is relevant to point out that the firing of PR neurons has been linearly correlated with the propagation of generalized seizure, possibly originated in other brain regions (11,13).

Another piece of interest is that PR cells exert a tonic (GABAergic) control upon DAergic cells of PC which, in turn, constitute the biological substrate for the reinforcing properties and craving of drugs of abuse (25,26). Thus, some BDZ receptor ligands might have abuse liability because of their disinhibitory action of DAergic cell firing. On the contrary, both inhibition of PR cells and excitation of PC cells by systemic ETH are unmodifiable by FLUM, suggesting that ETH does not directly interfere with BDZ recognition sites. However, the inhibition of PR cell firing as well as the behavioral and EEG changes by moderate doses of ETH can be reverted by analeptic drugs such as GABA antagonists (picrotoxin and bicuciline), excitatory β-CBs (DMCM, β-CCM), and excitatory BDZs (Ro 15-4513), all drugs which ultimately reduce the GABA-gated Cl⁻ conductance (2,5,6,14,20,42,44).

ACKNOWLEDGMENTS

We would like to thank Stefano Aramo for the experimental assistance, and Gabriela Martin for the word processing.

We are also grateful to Dr. Stefano Vicini and Dr. Janie Smith for their comments on the manuscript.

REFERENCES

1. Araki, M., McGeer, P.L. and McGeer, E.G. (1985): Brain Research, 331: 17-24.
2. Barnard, E.A. and Seeburg, P.H. (1988): In: Chloride Channels and Their Modulation by Neurotransmitters and Drugs, Adv. Biochem. Psychopharmacol., Vol. 45, Biggio, G. and Costa, E., eds., Raven Press, New York, pp. 1-18.
3. Biggio, G., Concas, A., Corda, A. and Serra, M. (1989): Eur. J. Pharmacol., 161: 173-180.
4. Biggio, G. and Costa, E. (1983): Benzodiazepine Recognition site Ligands, Adv. in Biochem. Psychopharmacol., Vol. 38, Raven Press, New York.
5. Biggio, G., Giorgi, O., Concas, A. and Corda, M.G. (1989): In: Down Regulation of the GABA$_A$ Receptor Complex Induced by Chronic Treatment with Its Allosteric Modulators, Fidia Research Foundation Symposium Series, Vol. 1, Barnard, E.A. and Costa, E., eds., Raven Press, New York, pp. 71-89.
6. Corda, M.G., Giorgi, O., Longoni, B., Fernandez, A. and Biggio, G. (1988): In: Chloride Channesl and Their Modulation by Neurotransmitters and Drugs, Adv. in Biochem. Psychopharmacol., Vol. 45, Biggio, G. and Costa, E., eds., Raven Press, New York, pp. 293-306.
7. Corda, M.G., Concas, A., Porceddu, E., Sanna, E. and Biggio, G. (1986): Neuropharmacology, 25: 59-62.
8. Corda, M.G., Giorgi, O., Longoni, B., Ongini, E., Montalto, S. and Biggio, G. (1988): Life Sciences, 42: 189-197.
9. Costa, E. and Guidotti, A. (1979): Ann. Rev. Pharmacol. Toxicol., 19: 531-545.
10. Dray, A. (1980): Progress in Neurobiology, 14/15: 221-336.
11. Gale, K. (1988): Epilepsia, 29, Suppl. 2: 515-534.
12. Gessa, G.L., Yoon, K-W.P., Boi, V., Westfall, T.C. and Mereu, G.P. (1986): Society for Neuroscience, 16th Annual Meeting, Abstract 133.17, Vol. 12/1, p. 486.
13. Gonzales, L.P. and Hettinger, M.K. (1984): Brain Research, 298: 163-166.

14. Grace, A.A. and Bunney, B.S. (1979): Eur. J. Pharmacol., 59: 211-218.
15. Haefely, W.E. (1983): In: Benzodiazepine Recognition Site Ligands, Adv. in Biochem. Psychopharmacol., Vol. 38, Biggio, G. and Costa, E., eds., Raven Press, New York, pp. 73-93.
16. Haefely, W.E. (1988): In: Chloride Channels and Their Modulation by Neurotransmitters and Drugs, Adv. in Biochemical. Psychopharmacol., Vol. 45, Biggio, G. and Costa, E., eds., Raven Press, New York, pp. 275-292.
17. Langer, S.Z., Arbilla, S., Scatton, B., Niddam, R. and Dubois, A. (1988): In: Imidazopyridines in Sleep Disorders, L.E.R.S. Monograph, Vol. 6, Sauvanet, J.P., Langer, S.Z. and Morselli, P.L., eds., Raven Press, New York, pp. 55-70.
18. Lo, M.M.S., Niehoff, D.L., Kuhar, M.J. and Snyder, S.H. (1983): Nature, 306: 57.
19. MacDonald, R.L. and Barker, J.L. (1979): Brain Research, 167: 323-336.
20. Marrosu, F., Carcangiu, G., Passino, N., Aramo, S. and Mereu, G. (1989): Synapse, 3: 117-128.
21. Mereu, G.P.: unpublished data.
22. Mereu, G. and Biggio, G. (1983): In: Benzodiazepine Recognition Site Ligands, Adv. in Biochem. Psychopharmacol., Vol. 38, Biggio, G. and Costa, E., eds., Raven Press, New York, pp. 201-209.
23. Mereu, G., Corda, G.P., Carcangiu, G.P., Giorgi, O. and Biggio, G. (1987): Life Sciences, 40: 1423-1430.
24. Mereu, G., Fadda, E. and Gessa, G.L. (1984): Brain Research, 292: 63-69.
25. Mereu, G. and Gessa, G.L. (1985): Brain Research, 360: 325-330.
26. Mereu, G.P., Passino, N., Carcangiu, G. and Gessa, G.L. (1988): In: Neurodegenerative Disorders, Nappi, G., Hornykiewicz, O., Agnoli, A., Fariello, R.G. and Clavazza, A., eds., Raven Press, New York, pp. 287-301.
27. Olsen, R.W. (1982): Ann. Rev. Pharmacol. Toxicol., 22: 245-277.
28. Passino, N., Peduto, V.A., Carcangiu, G.P., Boi, V. and Mereu, G.P. (1987): Society for Neuroscience, 17th Annual Meeting, 1987, Abstract n.253.4, Vol. 13/2, p. 913.
29. Polc, P., Bonetti, E.P., Schaffner, R. and Haefely, W. (1982): Naunyn Schmiedburg's Arch. Pharmacol., 321: 260-264.
30. Pritchett, D.B., Luddens, L. and Seeburg, P.H. (1989): Science, 245: 1389-1392.
31. Puia, G., Santi, M.R., Vicini, S., Pritchett, D.B., Seeburg, P.H. and Costa, E. (1989): Proc. Natl. Acad. Sci., USA, 86: 7275-7279.
32. Ribak, E.C., Vaughn, J.E., Daito, K., Barber, R. and Roberts, E. (1976): Brain Research, 116: 287-298.

33. Richards, J.G., Glintz, R., Schoch, P. and Mohler, H. (1988): In: Chloride Channels and Their Modulation by Neurotransmitters and Drugs, Adv. in Biochem. Psychopharmacol., Vol. 45, Biggio, G. and Costa, E., eds., Raven Press, New York, pp. 27-46.

34. Ross, R.J., Waszczak, B.L., Lee, E.K. and Walters, J.R. (1982): Life Siences, 31: 1025-1035.

35. Sanger, D.J. and Zikovic, B. (1987): Neuropharmacology, 26: 1513-1518.

36. Santi, M.R., Cox, D.H. and Guidotti, A. (1988): J. Neurochemistry, 50/4: 1080-1085.

37. Sequier, J.M., Richards, J.G., Malherbe, P., Price, G.W., Mathews, S. and Mohler, H. (1988): Proc Natl. Acad. Sci. USA, 85: 7815-7819.

38. Sieghart, W. (1988): In: Imidazopyridines in Sleep Disorders, L.E.R.S. Monograph, Vol. 6, Sauvanet, J.P., Langer, S.Z. and Morselli, P.L., eds., Raven Press, New York, pp. 39-45.

39. Suzdak, P.D., Glowa, J.R., Crawley, J.N., Schwartz, R.D., Skolnick, P. and Paul, S.M. (1986): Science 234: 1243-1247.

40. Tallman, J. (1988): In: Chloride Channels and Their Modulation by Neurotransmitters and Drugs, Adv. in Biochem. Psychopharmacol., Vol. 45, Biggio, G. and Costa, E., eds., Raven Press, New York, pp. 19-25.

41. Toussi, H.R., Schatz, R.A. and Waszczak. B.L. (1987): Eur. J. Pharmacol., 137: 261-264.

42. Vicini, S. Mienville, J.-M. and Costa, E. (1987): J. Pharmacol. Exp. Therap. 243: 1195-1201.

43. Waszczak, B.L. (1983): Neuropharmacology, 22/8: 953-959.

44. Waszczak, B.L. Eng, N. and Walters, J.R. (1980): Brain Research, 188: 185-197.

45. Waszczak, B.L., Lee, E.K. and Walters, J.R. (1986): J. Pharmacol Exp. Therap., 239: 606-611.

46. Waszczak, B.L. and Walters, J.R. (1986): J. Neurosci., 6: 120-126.

47. Wilson, M.A. and Gallager, D.W. (1989): J. Pharmacol Exp. Therap., 248: 886-891 .

GABA and Benzodiazepine Receptor Subtypes,
edited by Giovanni Biggio and Erminio Costa.
Raven Press, New York © 1990.

GABA$_B$ RECEPTORS AND THEIR HETEROGENEITY

N G Bowery, C Knott, R Moratalla & G D Pratt
Department of Pharmacology, The School of Pharmacy,
29/39 Brunswick Square London WC1N 1AX.

Two receptors subtypes for the neurotransmitter GABA, GABA$_A$ and GABA$_B$, are now firmly established however the full extent of any heterogeneity within each of these classes has yet to be realized. Evidence has accrued over a number of years to indicate the possible separation of bicuculline-sensitive GABA$_A$ receptors into subclasses based on their location, ligand affinity and relative sensitivities to bicuculline (1,2,4,10,12,21,29,32,36,40,48). Recently this has culminated in a separation based on the multiple α, β & γ subunit sequences of cloned cDNA's for the GABA$_A$ receptor (42,45,47). In situ hybridization studies in mammalian brain indicate that GABA$_A$ receptors formed from separate receptor subunits have different locations and these may have separate physiological roles. However distinct functional properties have yet to be ascertained for the subunits and their subclasses even though each subunit may convey a specific property to the GABA$_A$ receptor complex. For example, the γ subunit may be responsible for conveying high-affinity benzodiazepine binding in the receptor complex.

Similar detailed analysis of the GABA$_B$ receptor has yet to be done and only tentative subclassification of this site thus far is implied from functional or binding assays. However, there are many reasons to believe that separate GABA$_B$ receptor subtypes do exist in spite of the lack of definitive pharmacological evidence. For example, GABA$_B$ receptor activation can either increase K$^+$ conductance or decrease Ca^{++} conductance in mammalian neurones and these effects can occur independently (13,15,18,19,27,28,39). However no pharmacological separation in these actions has been demonstrated.

Separate receptor binding sites have also been suggested on the basis of the Hill coefficients for the displacement of radiolabelled baclofen binding to $GABA_B$ sites in mammalian brain membranes (43) but again the data are insufficient for receptors exhibiting distinct properties to be defined from these observations alone. Recent studies, on the neurochemistry of $GABA_B$ receptor activation and the pharmacology of the pre- and postsynaptic responses to $GABA_B$ receptor activation in hippocampal slices (discussed below) have provided stronger evidence but even with these experiments more data are still required before we can truly assign separate receptor classifications.

$GABA_B$ sites and cyclic AMP generation

Separate neurochemical responses to $GABA_B$ receptor activation associated with cAMP generation in brain tissue have become established. Firstly, enhancement of hormone-stimulated cAMP accumulation in slices and secondly, inhibition of basal as well as forskolin-stimulated cAMP formation in membranes as well as slices (23,24,25,30,31,51,53) (Fig 1). An additional biochemical effect, inhibition of 5HT-and histamine-induced phosphatidylinositol metabolism, has been observed in certain species (11,20) but little significance can be attached to this effect at present. The enhancement of β-adrenoceptor -mediated cAMP formation produced by $GABA_B$ site activation may be mediated through the action of phospholipase A_2 since inhibitors of this enzyme prevent the response to GABA or baclofen (31). However phospholipase A_2 inhibition does not affect the inhibitory action of GABA or baclofen on cAMP formation.

The inhibitory action of GABA and baclofen on cAMP formation can be prevented by prior treatment with pertussis toxin (53) which is known to ADP-ribosylate G-proteins associated with certain receptor-effector coupling mechanisms (33). Whether a similar G-protein coupling can also be implicated in the enhancement of cAMP formation by $GABA_B$ site activation is unclear. Our experimental data suggest that a G_i/G_o - protein is not involved. Adult rats were injected intrahippocampally (coordinates 3.0, 2.0, -3.5) with pertussis toxin (4 ug) 3-8 days

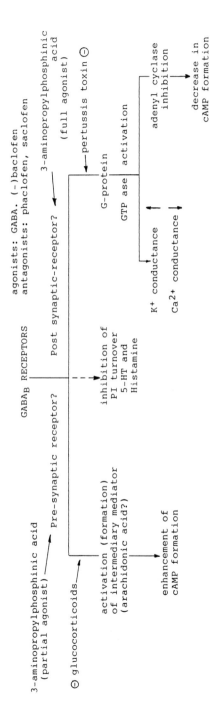

Fig 1 Summary of possible second messenger systems attributed to GABA_B receptor activation in mammalian brain

prior to the preparation of hippocampal slices. This failed to prevent the stimulation of cAMP formation by noradrenaline or the ability of baclofen to enhance the response to the catecholamine (8). In slices from the same animals the inhibition of forskolin-stimulated cAMP accumulation was completely blocked and the activation of GTPase activity, which accompanies $GABA_B$-mediated inhibition of cAMP formation, was also inhibited.

The lack of effect of pertussis toxin on the enhancement of cAMP formation was not observed by Wojcik et al (52) . These authors have reported that both the inhibition and enhancement were reduced in cerebral cortex slices 4 days after i.c.v. injection of 6ug pertussis toxin. Unfortunately the reasons for this disparity are unclear although a different brain region was used.

Irrespective of the possible G-protein involvement a separation of these two systems now appears to be emerging based on the selectivities of certain GABA and baclofen analogues for each effect. 3-aminopropylphosphinic acid is a new selective $GABA_B$ agonist (6,14,41, see also 26) with a binding affinity approximately 100 fold higher than GABA or baclofen. This compound inhibits forskolin-stimulated cAMP in the same manner producing the same maximum inhibition as baclofen. However, whilst it also mimics baclofen in enhancing cAMP formation in the presence of noradrenaline it fails to produce the same maximum response as baclofen. The enhancement is only 50% of maximum (Fig 2). Thus 3-aminopropylphosphinic acid appears to be a partial agonist in this system. This conclusion is supported by additional experiments in which we have observed that a supramaximal concentration of 3-aminopropylphosphinic acid will inhibit responses to the full agonist baclofen (Fig 2) (41). This would suggest that the site associated with enhancement of cAMP levels is distinct from that responsible for inhibition of adenylate cyclase.

In a recent report by Scherer et al (44) data are provided showing that 3-aminopropylphosphinic acid, which has affinity for $GABA_B$ binding sites and inhibits forskolin-stimulated cAMP accumulation, does not affect the response to β-adrenoceptor activation. The authors conclude that subsets of $GABA_B$ receptors are responsible for these separate effects.

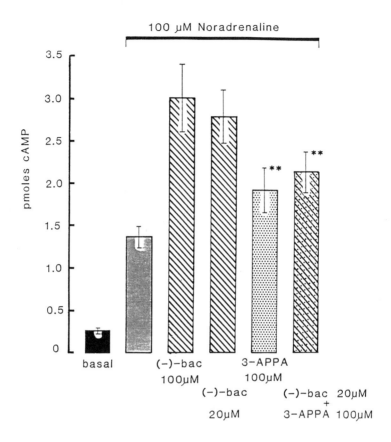

Fig 2
Comparison of the effects of (-)baclofen ((-)bac) and
3-aminopropylphosphinic acid (3-APPA) on the level of
cAMP in rat cerebral cortex slices produced by
noradrenaline (100μM). Generation of cAMP was
measured as described by Hill (23). The data derive
from 5 separate experiments performed in triplicate.
The amount of cAMP generated by 100μM noradrenaline
alone (▓) was maximal and 100μM (-)-baclofen (▨)
produced the maximum enhancement in this response.
3-aminopropylphosphinic acid (3-APPA ▨) failed to
produce the same level of enhancement. Combination
of (-)-baclofen (20μM) and 3-APPA (100μM) (▨)
produced less enhancement than (-)-baclofen alone.
Neither (-)-baclofen nor 3-APPA in the absence of
noradrenaline produced any effect on cAMP levels.

We have observed the converse effect, enhancement of the noradrenaline effect with no inhibition of the response to forskolin with [c(4-chlorophenyl)5-fluoro 2-hydroxy benzilidene amino]-4-butanoate solution (SL75102). This compound is a $GABA_B$ agonist with an affinity of 0.5uM (cf GABA 80nM) for $GABA_B$ binding sites in rat brain membranes (7) . However at concentrations up to 1 mM it failed to inhibit the action of forskolin on cAMP formation whereas it did produce enhancement of the response to noradrenaline.

Pre- and post-synaptic separation of $GABA_B$ sites?

The association of $GABA_B$ sites with G-protein(s) is not confined to biochemical studies. Electrophysiological experiments have shown a clear link in many brain regions as well as in dorsal root ganglia where the stable GTP analogue GTP S has been shown to augment the decrease in Ca^{++} conductance elicited by GABA and baclofen (46). In rat hippocampal slices $GABA_B$ site activation of pyramidal cells produces an increase in membrane K^+ conductance (3,16,19,27,28,39). This effect is blocked by phaclofen, the selective $GABA_B$ antagonist (34). Moreover the late inhibitory post synaptic potential recorded in CA1 cells following stimulation of the stratum radiatum is also blocked by phaclofen implicating $GABA_B$ sites as the mediator of this synaptic potential (16,49). The late ipsp can also be prevented by pretreatment in vivo with pertussis toxin (50). By contrast, the fast ipsp, which precedes the $GABA_B$ ipsp, is unaffected by pertussis toxin treatment. This synaptic potential is mediated through bicuculline-sensitive $GABA_A$ receptors.

A recent report Dutar & Nicoll (17, see also ref 22) indicate that there are two components of the $GABA_B$ response to baclofen on hippocampal CA1 cells. They suggest that baclofen acts presynaptically to reduce the release of excitatory transmitter from terminals innervating the CA1 cells, which arise from the commissural and Schaffer collateral pathways. Baclofen also acts postsynaptically to hyperpolarize the pyramidal cells. Pertussis toxin pretreatment prevented the latter response but failed to alter the presynaptic response to baclofen. In addition phaclofen blocked the postsynaptic but not the presynaptic response whereas the phorbol ester, phorbol-12,13-dibutyrate reduced both responses. It was concluded that separate receptors mediate the pre-and post-synaptic response.

We are currently attempting to demonstrate this apparent separation by neurochemistry and receptor autoradiography. Unfortunately preliminary data from autoradiographical studies provide no support for the electrophysiological separation found in the CA1 area. Binding to $GABA_B$ sites on neuronal membranes is reduced by pertussis toxin pretreatment (5) and similarly injection of pertussis toxin intrahippocampally reduced the binding of ^{3}H-GABA to hippocampal regions in rat brain sections (Fig 3).

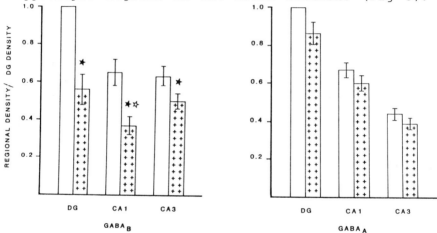

Fig 3
Effect of intrahippocampal pertussis toxin injection on the density of $GABA_A$ and $GABA_B$ binding in hippocampal regions of rat brain slices. Pertussis toxin (4µg) was injected into the right hippocampal CA1 region of 6 rats. After 4 days 10um cryostat sections were prepared and $GABA_A$ and $GABA_B$ sites labelled with 3HGABA (50nM) as described previously (9). Regional binding densities were determined from autoradiograms by image analysis and the values expressed as a ratio of the density in the untreated dentate gyrus. Values were determined from 22 sections each for GABAA and GABAB binding. Open histogram bars represent mean values obtained from the untreated hippocampus. The bars with crosses represent values from pertussis-toxin treated hippocampus. CA1 and CA3 measurements were made in stratum radiatum. The ordinate value of 1 for GABAB and GABAA represents 1552 and 3178 nCi/g tissue respectively (calibration with Amersham International Microscales).
* indicates significant difference from untreated side ($p < 0.05$)
** indicates significant difference compared with change in CA3 region.

In particular, binding in CA1 was reduced by 43%. However it was noted in this study that binding within the CA3 region was much less reduced (21%)

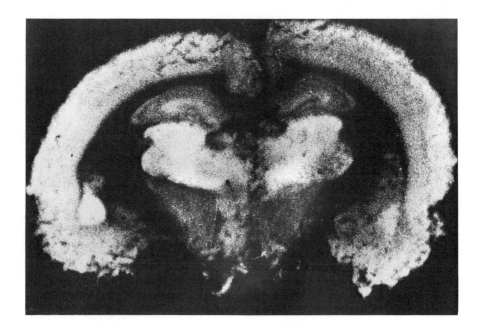

Fig 4
Effect of in vitro incubation with pertussis toxin on
GABA_B binding in a rat brain section. Coronal 250μm
sections from the same rat brain were bisected along
the midline and incubated for 24 hours at 25°C in
Krebs- bicarbonate buffer with or without pertussis
toxin (10μM). After this period the half sections
were mounted together on cork chucks and 10uM
cryostat sections prepared. GABA_B site labelling was
then performed as described previously (9) and the
autoradiograms obtained by apposition to Hyperfilm
for 4 weeks. A colour-coded image of the
autoradiogram is shown to highlight the regional
differences.

than in the CA1 region even though ventral and dorsal CA1 regions were equally affected. This suggested that limited diffusion may not account for the difference in binding between CA1 and CA3. Since the Schaffer collaterals derive from CA3 cells the weaker effect of pertussis toxin on the binding in this region might be due to a predominance of 'pre-synaptic type' receptor on the cell bodies whereas in the CA1 region pertussis toxin-sensitive 'postsynaptic type' receptor binding predominates.

We have assessed the contribution of poor diffusion possibly accounting for the differential effect of pertussis toxin by incubating brain slices in the toxin in vitro. Coronal blocks, <400 μm thick, of fresh brain were incubated for up to 24 hours at 25°C in Krebs bicarbonate buffer containing pertussis toxin, 10μM (Porton Products Ltd.) and NAD, ATP, thymidine, EDTA, dithiothreitol and $MgCl_2$. To compare untreated and toxin treated tissue each block was hemisected in the vertical plane and one half was incubated in pertussis toxin-free medium whilst the other half was incubated for the same period in toxin-containing medium. After incubation the half blocks were mounted together on cork chucks and rapidly frozen for the preparation of cryostat sections (10 μm). $GABA_B$ (and $GABA_A$) receptor autoradiography was then performed as previously described (9). Autoradiograms were obtained by apposing sections to Hyperfilm for 4 weeks.

Whilst pertussis toxin does not readily penetrate cells in vitro our preliminary experiments indicated a 25-30% reduction in the density of $GABA_B$ binding sites within the hippocampus after 24 hours incubation in 10 uM toxin (Fig 4). However the reduction in binding in the CA3 region was the same as within the CA1 (Table 1) which would suggest that limited diffusion may have accounted for the apparent difference observed in CA1 and CA3 after in vivo administration. Further in vitro and in vivo experiments are required to validate this conclusion.

Interestingly, the in vitro data shown in Table 1 indicate that binding in the caudate putamen is resistant to pertussis toxin. The majority of binding within this region also appears to be on presynaptic terminals since chronic lesions of the nigrostriatal and corticostriatal pathways produced a marked reduction in $GABA_B$ binding (37,38) whereas

Effect of Pertussis toxin (24h) in vitro on GABA$_B$
binding density in rat brain sections

Region	Control	Pertussis toxin	% Change
Cerebral Cortex Outer	19.9 ± .46	14.5 ± 1.0 *	-27
Cerebral Cortex Inner	13.3 ± .39	10.3 ± 0.5 *	-23
Caudate putamen	5.1 ± .29	5.1 ± .28	0
Hippocampus CA1	6.5 ± .36	4.3 ± .40 *	-35
" CA3	7.3 ± .38	5.2 ± .49 *	-29
" Stratum Lucidum	10.5 ± .92	6.7 ± .59 *	-36
Dentate gyrus	10.4 ± .56	6.9 ± .47 *	-33
Cerebellum molecular layer	20.0 ± .98	9.9 ± 1.2 *	-50
Dorsolateral geniculate	18.5 ± 1.2	13.0 ± 1.9 *	-30
Medial geniculate body	18.9 ± 1.2	16.3 ± 2.3	-14
Corpus callosum	1.4 ± .17	1.4 ± .20	0

* p<.01

Table 1

Values indicate the mean density ± s.e.m (nCi/g
tissue) of GABA$_B$ binding sites in 11 brain regions
determined from 27 sections (3 rat brains). The
control and pertussis toxin values derive from the
same brain sections, one half incubated for 24h in
Krebs-bicarbonate buffer alone, the other half in
buffer containing pertussis toxin (10μM) for the same
time. Values were determined by reference to tritium
standards (Amersham International) on the same
films.

kainic acid injection into the striatum produced little or no change (35). This apparent insensitivity to pertussis toxin of a predominately presynaptic site may provide an important model for studying the pharmacological characteristics of the pre- as compared to the postsynaptic receptor.

In conclusion we have so far been unable to confirm the electrophysiological evidence for a separation between pre- and post-synaptic GABA$_B$ binding sites within the rat hippocampus using pertussis toxin. Nevertheless we would support a receptor separation based on the pharmacology of the GABA$_B$-induced changes in cAMP levels. However our data are still preliminary and further experimentation is required.

ACKNOWLEDGEMENT

Financial support by the Medical Research Council is gratefully acknowledged.

REFERENCES

1   Alger BE & Nicoll RA. (1982) J. Physiol. Lond., 328, 125-141.
2   Allan RD, Evans RH & Johnston GAR. (1980) Br. J. Pharmacol., 70, 609-615.
3   Andrade R, Malenka MC & Nicoll RA. (1986) Science, 234, 1261-1265.
4   Arbilla S, Kanal L & Langer SZ. (1979) Eur. J. Pharmacol., 57, 211-217.
5   Asano T, Ui M & Ogasawara N. (1985) J. Biol. Chem, 260, 12653-12658.
6   Bittiger H, Reymann N, Hall R & Kane P. (1988) Eur. Neurosc. Assoc. Proc., September.
7   Bowery NG, Hill DR & Hudson AL. (1982) Neuropharmacol., 21, 391-395.
8   Bowery NG, Hill DR & Moratalla R. (1989) In: Allosteric modulation of amino acid receptors: therapeutic implications. Eds: EA Barnard & E Costa. pp 159-172. Raven Press, New York.
9   Bowery NG, Hudson AL & Price GW. (1987) Neuroscience, 20, 365-385.
10 Brennan, MJW. (1982) J. Neurochem., 38, 264-266.
11 Crawford MLA, Young JM. (1988) J. Neurochem., 51, 1441-1447.

12   Curtis DR. (1978) In: Amino acids as chemical
     transmitters. Ed F Fonnum. pp 55-86. Plenum
     Press, New York.
13   Desarmenien M, Feltz P, Occhipinti G, Santangelo
     F & Schlichter R. (1984) Br. J. Pharmacol., 81,
     327-333.
14   Dingwall JG, Ehrenfreund J, Hall RG & Jack J.
     (1987) Phosphorus and Sulfur, 30, 571-575.
15   Dolphin AC & Scott RH. (1986) Br. J.
     Pharmacol., 88, 213-220.
16   Dutar P & Nicoll, RA. (1988) Nature, 332, 156-
     158.
17   Dutar P & Nicoll RA. (1988) Neuron, 1, 585-598.
18   Feltz A, Demeneix B, Feltz P, Taleb O, Trouslard
     J, Bossu J-L & Dupont J-L. (1987) Biochimie, 69,
     395-406.
19   Gahwiler BH & Brown DA. (1985) Proc. Natl.
     Acad. Sci. USA. 82, 1558-1562.
20   Godfrey PP, Grahame-Smith DG & Gray JA. (1988)
     Eur. J. Pharmacol., 152, 185-188.
21   Guidotti A, Gale K, Suria A, Toffano G. (1979)
     Brain Res., 172, 566-571.
22   Harrison NL, Large GD & Barker JL. (1988)
     Neurosci. Lett., 85, 105-109.
23   Hill DR. (1985) Br. J. Pharmacol., 84, 249-257
24   Hill DR, Bowery NG & Hudson AL. (1984)
     J. Neurochem., 42, 652-657.
25   Hill DR, Moratalla R & Bowery NG. (1989) In:
     GABA, basic research and clinical applications.
     Eds: NG Bowery & G Nistico. pp 224-238.
     Pythagora, Rome,
26   Hills JM, Dingsdale RA, Parsons ME, Dolle RE &
     Howson W. (1989) Br. J. Pharmacol., 97, 1292-
     1296.
27   Inoue M, Matsuo T & Ogata N. (1985) Br. J.
     Pharmacol., 84, 833-842.
28   Inoue M, Matsuo T & Ogata N. (1985) Br. J.
     Pharmacol., 84, 843-852.
29   Johnston GAR. (1981) In: The role of peptides
     and amino acids as neurotransmitters. Alan R
     Liss, pp 1-17, New York.
30   Karbon EW & Enna SJ. (1985) Mol. Pharmacol., 27,
     53-59.
31   Karbon EW & Enna SJ. (1989) In: GABA, basic
     research and clinical applications. Eds: NG
     Bowery & G Nistico. pp 205-223, Pythagora Press,
     Rome.
32   Karobath M, Placheta P, Lippitsch M & Krogsgaard
     Larsen P. (1979) Nature, Lond., 278, 748-749.
33   Katada T & Ui M. (1982) Proc. Natl. Acad. Sci.
     USA, 79, 3129-3133.

34   Kerr DIB, Ong J, Prager RH, Gynther BD & Curtis
      DR. (1987) Brain Res., 405, 150-154.
35   Kilpatrick GJ, Muhyaddin MS, Roberts PJ, &
      Woodruff GN. (1983) Br. J. Pharmac., 78,
      suppl., 6P.
36   Mitchell PR & Martin IL. (1978) Nature, Lond.,
      274, 904-905.
37   Moratalla R, Barth T & Bowery NG. (1989)
      Neuropharmacology. (in press).
38   Moratalla R & Bowery NG. (1988) Br. J.
      Pharmacol., 95, 476P.
39   Newberry NR, Nicoll RA. (1985) J. Physiol.,
      360, 161-185.
40   Nistri A & Constanti A. (1979) Prog.
      Neurobiol., 13, 117-235.
41   Pratt GD, Knott C, Davey R & Bowery NG. (1989)
      Br. J. Pharmacol., 96, 141P.
42   Pritchett DB, Sontheimer H, Shivers BD, Ymer S,
      Kettenmenn HK, Schofield PR & Seeburg PH.
      (1989) Nature, 338, 582-585.
43   Robinson TN, Stirling JM, Cross AJ & Green AR.
      (1988) Neurochem. Int., 13, Suppl, 1, 165,
      F257.
44   Scherer RW, Ferkany JW & Enna SJ. (1988) Brain
      Research Bull., 21, 439-443.
45   Schofield PR, Darlison MG, Fujita N, Burt DR,
      Stephenson FA, Rodriquez H, Rhee LM,
      Ramachandran J, Reale V, Glencorse TA, Seeburg
      PH & Barnard EA. (1987) Nature, 328, 221-227.
46   Scott RH & Dolphin AC. (1986) Neurosci. Lett.,
      69, 59-64.
47   Sequier JM, Richards JG, Malherbe P, Price GW,
      Matthews S & Mohler H. (1988) Proc. Natl. Acad.
      Sci. USA., 85, 7815-7819.
48   Snodgrass SR. (1978) Nature, Lond., 274, 392-
      394.
49   Soltesz I, Haby M, Leresche N & Crunelli V.
      (1988) Brain Res., 448, 351-354.
50   Thalmann, RH. (1988) J. Neurosci., 8, 4589-
      4602.
51   Wojcik WJ & Neff NH. (1984) Mol. Pharmacol.,
      25, 24-28.
52   Wojcik WJ, Paez X & Ulivi M. (1989) In:
      Allosteric modulation of amino acid receptors:
      therapeutic implications. Eds EA Barnard & E
      Costa. pp 173-193. Raven Press, New York.
53   Xu J & Wojcik WJ. (1986) J. Pharmac. Exp.
      Ther., 239, 568-573.

GABA and Benzodiazepine Receptor Subtypes,
edited by Giovanni Biggio and Erminio Costa.
Raven Press, New York © 1990.

GABA$_A$ AND GABA$_B$ RECEPTOR PHARMACOLOGY IN CULTURED SPINAL CORD NEURONS

M.K. Ticku, A.K. Mehta and G.L. Kamatchi

Department of Pharmacology
The University of Texas Health Science Center at San Antonio
7703 Floyd Curl Drive
San Antonio, Texas 78284-7764 USA

GABA receptors are widely distributed in the CNS and are involved in modulating CNS excitability both pre- and post-synaptically. Historically, GABA receptors have been classified into two subtypes, viz GABA$_A$ receptors that are activated by GABA agonists like muscimol, and the responses are blocked by bicuculline and facilitated by benzodiazepine (BZ) agonists and barbiturates (e.g., 4), and GABA$_B$ receptors that are activated by baclofen, their responses are blocked by phaclofen, and these receptors are coupled to voltage-gated Ca^{2+} channels, K$^+$-channels, and/or G-proteins (5,9,12,28,36). However, recent cloning data indicates that GABA$_A$ receptor composition may be highly diverse in terms of subunit composition and distribution in the CNS (e.g., 31; Seeburg this volume). Radioligand binding studies have demonstrated the subunits, that form the GABA$_A$ receptor complex, having multiple allosteric binding sites for GABA agonists, BZs, picrotoxin-like convulsants, barbiturates, and steroids (29,35).

Our laboratory over the years has developed cultured spinal cord neurons to study GABA synaptic pharmacology _in_ _vitro_. This chapter describes some of our recent studies characterizing GABA$_A$ receptor pharmacology using ^{36}Cl-influx assay, and GABA$_B$ pharmacology using depolarization-induced (Ca^{2+}-activated) ^{86}Rb-efflux in these neurons (3,14,33).

METHODS

Cell Culture

Spinal cords from 13-14 day-old C57Bl/6J mouse embryos were removed, minced, dissociated and plated on poly-L-lysine-coated sterile coverslips, as described (16). The neurons were grown in culture for 7-8 days.

^{36}Cl-Influx

^{36}Cl-influx was measured as described previously (16,23,25). Briefly, coverslips containing neurons were transferred to physiological buffer containing ^{36}Cl (2 µci/ml) in the absence and presence of various drugs. The influx was terminated after 5 sec, as described earlier (23).

^{86}Rb-Efflux

Coverslips containing neurons were incubated with ^{86}Rb (2 µci/ml) overnight, as described (14). Prior to initiating efflux, the coverslips were washed four times with 2 ml each of non-depolarizing buffer (in mM: NaCl 145, KCl 5, MgCl$_2$ 2, CaCl$_2$ 1.8, HEPES 10, and glucose 10, adjusted to pH 7.4 with trisbase) to remove excess ^{86}Rb. The efflux was initiated by incubating the coverslips for a 30 sec period in petri dishes containing depolarizing buffer (100 mM KCl substituted for an equal amount of NaCl) in the absence and presence of baclofen and other drugs. The efflux was terminated, and % ^{86}Rb-efflux was estimated as described earlier (3,14,33).

RESULTS AND DISCUSSION

GABA$_A$ Receptor-Induced ^{36}Cl-Influx

The cultured spinal cord neurons used in the present study exhibit a high affinity Na$^+$-dependent [^{3}H]GABA uptake mechanism, which was sensitive to nipecotic acid, β-alanine, low Na$^+$, and temperature (16). These results suggest the presence of GABAergic presynaptic nerve terminals in these cultures. Binding studies to intact cells indicated the presence of specific and saturable [^{3}H]flunitrazepam binding (16,22). The specific [^{3}H]flunitrazepam binding was inhibited by BZ agonists, antagonist flumazenil (Ro 15-1788), β-carbolines, and enhanced by GABA agonists and other sedative-hypnotics that inhibit picrotoxin binding such as etazolate, (+)etomidate, and pentobarbital (22). The enhancing effect of GABA agonists was blocked by bicuculline and picrotoxin. These results indicate the presence of GABA, BZ, picrotoxin, and barbiturate sites in the cultured spinal cord neurons. Developmental studies indicated that BZ receptors, GABA enhancement of BZ binding, GABA-gated Cl$^-$-channels, and bicuculline antagonism can be observed in spinal cord cultured neurons as early as three days following plating in vitro (24).

The functional coupling of GABA$_A$ receptors to Cl-channels was demonstrated by the ability of GABA and other GABA$_A$ agonists to increase ^{36}Cl-influx. GABA (K$_m$ = 9 µM) and muscimol (K$_m$ = 2 µM) produced a concentration-dependent increase in ^{36}Cl-influx (16,23). The enhancing effect of GABA was blocked in a concentration-dependent manner by bicuculline and picrotoxin (16). Basal, but not GABA-stimulated, ^{36}Cl-influx was inhibited by Cl$^-$-HCO$_3^-$ exchange inhibitor, DIDS and

Na^+-Cl^- co-transport inhibitor, furosemide (16). Further, GABA-induced ^{36}Cl-influx was neuronal, since conditions that favor non-neuronal cell-growth did not exhibit an increase in ^{36}Cl-influx induced by GABA (16). Glycine also activated Cl^--channels in the spinal cord neurons, however, these channels are distinct from GABA-gated Cl^--channels, since the effect of glycine and GABA were additive.

TABLE 1. <u>Potencies and efficacies for enhancement or inhibi-</u><u>tion of the GABA-induced ^{36}Cl-influx by BZs and</u> <u>beta-carbolines in spinal cord neurons</u>

Drug	EC_{50}	IC_{50}	E_{max}
	nM		%
Flunitrazepam	133 ± 18		101 ± 8
Clonazepam	175 ± 7		88 ± 6
Diazepam	450 ± 29		101 ± 10
Flurazepam	1,500 ± 282		85 ± 7
Ro 15-1788	3,900 ± 458		62 ± 3
DMCM		6 ± 1.4	-69 ± 8
Beta-CCE		21 ± 4	-60 ± 4
Ro 15-4513		1,200 ± 141	-49 ± 5
FG 7142		2,850 ± 910	-43 ± 6

Values are means ± S.E. of two to five experiments, each performed using three coverslips. Reproduced with permission from (25).

Benzodiazepine and βeta-Carboline Modulation of GABA_A Receptor-Induced ^{36}Cl-Influx

Table 1 summarizes the effect of BZ agonists, flumazenil (Ro 15-1788), beta carboline, and other inverse agonists on GABA-induced ^{36}Cl-influx in cultured spinal cord neurons (25). BZ agonists produced a concentration-dependent increase in GABA (10 μM)-induced ^{36}Cl-influx with the following potency rank order: flunitrazepam > clonazepam > diazepam >> flurazepam. While clonazepam and flurazepam gave slightly lower maximal enhancing effect (E_{max}), our studies were unable to determine if these drugs acted as partial agonists (see 25), as suggested by others (7). The BZ agonists like diazepam and flunitrazepam shifted the GABA dose-response curve to the left and decreased the K_m value of GABA from 10 to 5 μM, without affecting the maximal response (Fig. 1). When GABA receptors were fully saturated with the agonist (100 μM GABA), BZ agonists did not produce any additional effect. These results are consistent with the notion that BZ agonists need ongoing

GABAergic activity to produce their pharmacological effects (30).

Inverse agonists of the BZ recognition site inhibited GABA-induced ^{36}Cl-influx (DMCM > β-CCE >> Ro 15-4513 > FG 7142). DMCM gave a maximal inhibition of ~ 70% (25). Flumazenil (Ro 15-1788) exhibited partial agonistic activity at concentration > 1 μM. However, at concentration ≤ 1 μM, flumazenil reversed both the enhancing effect of diazepam and the inhibitory effect of DMCM (25). These results are consistent with the expected pharmacology of BZ agonist and inverse agonists and their relationship to GABA$_A$ergic transmission.

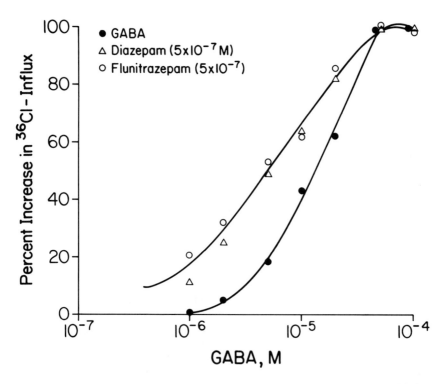

FIG. 1. Concentration-dependent increase by GABA on ^{36}Cl-influx in the absence and presence of diazepam and flunitrazepam. Values are means of a typical experiment (three coverslips), which was replicated twice with similar results. Reproduced with permission from (25).

Ethanol and GABA-Induced ^{36}Cl-Influx

Several lines of behavioral and pharmacological studies have implicated GABA$_A$ receptor system in the actions of ethanol (e.g., 11,17,34). This is also supported by some electrophysiological studies (6,8,26,27), however, contradictory reports have appeared (21). Recent electrophysiological studies have indicated a role for N-methyl-D-aspartate (NMDA) receptors in the actions of ethanol (18,19).

Ethanol has been shown to potentiate GABA-induced ^{36}Cl-influx in microsacs (1), neurosynaptosomes (32), and spinal cord neurons (23). Table 2 shows that in cultured spinal cord neurons, ethanol up to 20 mM does not alter the basal values,

TABLE 2. Direct effect of ethanol on ^{36}Cl-influx in cultured spinal cord neurons

Ethanol	% Increase Overall Basal
20 mM	2.5 ± 1.9 (n = 9)
50 mM	34.3 ± 3.9[a] (n = 9)
100 mM	37.1 ± 6.9[a] (n = 3)
500 mM	38.5 ± 3.1[a] (n = 3)

Coverslips with attached cells were washed twice in physiological buffer, before incubation with ethanol and ^{36}Cl for 10 sec, as described under "Methods." Values represent the mean ± S.D. of number of experiments indicated in the parenthesis. [a]P < 0.001, as compared to 20 mM ethanol. Reproduced with permission from (23).

whereas at higher concentrations (50-500 mM), ethanol gave a direct effect in the absence of GABA (23). The direct effect of ethanol was not concentration-dependent, but was blocked by bicuculline, picrotoxin, and inverse agonists of the BZ receptor site like Ro 15-4513 and FG 7142 (23).

For further characterization of ethanol enhancement of GABA$_A$ergic responses, a concentration of 20 mM was used. This concentration of ethanol increased the effect of submaximal concentration of GABA from 40 to 70% (Fig. 2). Furthermore, the ethanol enhancing effect of GABA responses was reversed by GABA antagonists like bicuculline and picrotoxin, and inverse agonists of the BZ recognition site, Ro 15-4513 and FG 7142 (23). The inhibitory effect of Ro 15-4513 on ethanol facilitation of GABA-induced ^{36}Cl-influx was reversed by Ro 15-1788, suggesting the involvement of central BZ recognition site in the action of Ro 15-4513. Like BZ agonists, ethanol (20 mM) shifted the GABA dose-response curve to the left without altering the maximal response. These results indicate that ethanol, at pharmacologically relevant concentrations, facilitates GABA$_A$ergic transmission. The exact site and the mechanism by which ethanol produces this facilitatory effect remains to be elucidated. Finally, since ethanol facilitates GABA$_A$ergic transmission and inhibits NMDA-mediated excitatory transmission (18,19) in the same concentration range (5-50 mM), both these receptor systems may be intimately involved in the actions of ethanol.

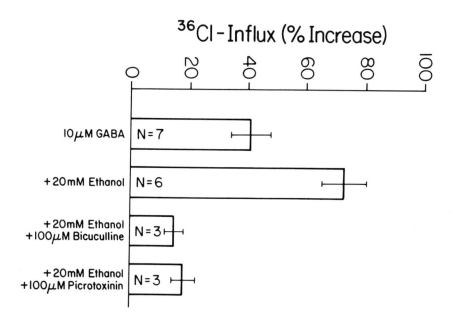

FIG. 2. Ethanol (20 mM) enhancement of GABA (10 μM)-induced ^{36}Cl-influx and its modification by GABA-receptor antagonists in cultured spinal cord neurons. Coverslips were preincubated with bicuculline and picrotoxin for 3 min before incubation with ^{36}Cl, GABA, and ethanol. Ethanol (20 mM) alone did not alter the basal values. The values represent mean ± S.E. of number of experiments indicated by "N." Basal values have been subtracted. Reproduced with permission from (23).

GABA$_B$ Receptor Pharmacology

GABA$_B$ receptor activation has been reported to decrease voltage-dependent Ca^{2+}-channels presynaptically (9,12), and activate K$^+$-channels postsynaptically (2,10). Involvement of adenylate cyclase and G-proteins in the effects of GABA$_B$ receptor stimulation has also been suggested (5,10,28,36). We have developed an assay to study presynaptic GABA$_B$ receptor pharmacology in cultured spinal cord neurons. This assay involves the effects of $GABA_B$ receptor stimulation on depolarization-induced Ca^{2+}-activated K^+-channels using ^{86}Rb-efflux (3,14). We have also described a similar assay for measuring $GABA_B$ responses in synaptosomes (33).

Table 3 shows that depolarizing concentration of K^+ increased ^{86}Rb-efflux from preloaded spinal cord neurons. This increase was inhibited by Ca^{2+}-channel blocker La^{3+} and agents which are known to block Ca^{2+}-activated K^+-channels, like TEA and quinine sulphate.

$GABA_B$ receptor specific agonist, (-)baclofen, inhibited the Ca^{2+}-activated ^{86}Rb-efflux in a concentration-dependent manner (Table 4). The inhibition was stereospecific and specific for $GABA_B$ receptor subtype, since phaclofen, a $GABA_B$ antagonist (15), reversed the (-)baclofen's effect (14). Since baclofen is known to inhibit voltage-gated Ca^{2+}-channels, the effect of baclofen can be attributed to this inhibitory effect on Ca^{2+}-channels.

Since previous studies have demonstrated the involvement of G-proteins in the baclofen's effects on Ca^{2+} current presynaptically (12) and K^+ conductance postsynaptically (2,10), we have investigated the effect of pertussis toxin in our system. Pertussis toxin treatment (140 ng/ml, overnight incubation) abolished the inhibitory effect of (-)baclofen on depolarization-induced ^{86}Rb-efflux (14). These results suggest that presynaptic $GABA_B$ receptors are coupled to G-proteins. However, a recent study has shown that baclofen's postsynaptic (slow IPSP), but not presynaptic effect in hippocampus was sensitive to pertussis toxin (10). In contrast, both the responses were blocked by the activator of protein kinase-C, phorbol ester. Table 5 shows that phorbol ester also blocks the inhibitory effect of (-)baclofen on ^{86}Rb-efflux in spinal cord neurons. Further, our studies have shown that forskolin, which activates protein kinase-A, also blocks (-)baclofen's effect (14).

These results are complex, and indicate that uncoupling of G-proteins by ADP ribosylation, and phosphorylation by either protein kinase-A or protein kinase-C, blocks depolarization-induced Ca^{2+}-activated ^{86}Rb-efflux. Effect of pertussis toxin to block $GABA_B$ responses could be attributed to the involvement of G-proteins in its actions (12). Since protein kinase-C can inactivate some G-proteins and/or phosphorylate receptors/channels (13), this may explain its effects on (-)baclofen responses. This observation is consistent with a previous report using hippocampal slice preparation (10). The effects of forskolin could be attributed to the coupling of $GABA_B$ receptors to adenylate cyclase (36). It may also be noted that elevation of cAMP can block Ca^{2+}-activated K^+-currents (20). However, it is also known that postsynaptic $GABA_B$ responses are cAMP-independent (20), but the involvement of cAMP in modulating presynaptic $GABA_B$ receptors is not clear.

TABLE 3. Effect of La^{3+}, TEA, and quinine sulfate on the depolarization-induced ^{86}Rb-efflux in spinal cord neurons

Treatment	% ^{86}Rb-Efflux (Mean ± S.D.)
5 mM KCl	5.03 ± 0.46
100 mM KCl	13.26 ± 0.75
100 mM KCl + 10^{-4} M La^{3+}	11.37 ± 1.11[a]
100 mM KCl + 2 X 10^{-4} M La^{3+}	8.98 ± 0.88[b]
100 mM KCl + 10^{-3} M TEA	7.12 ± 0.96[b]
100 mM KCl + 10^{-5} M quinine sulfate	8.50 ± 0.15[b]

The depolarization-induced ^{86}Rb-efflux was obtained with 100 mM KCl for 30 s, as described (14). Two coverslips were used for each treatment, as described in "Methods." The results are mean ± S.D. of four experiments.
[a] $P < 0.02$; [b] $P < 0.001$, as compared to 100 mM KCl. Reproduced with permission from (14).

TABLE 4. Concentration-dependent inhibition of ^{86}Rb-efflux by (-)baclofen in spinal cord neurons

Treatment	% ^{86}Rb-Efflux (Mean ± S.D.)
5 mM KCl	5.59 ± 0.42
100 mM KCl	16.00 ± 0.72
100 mM KCl + 10^{-6} M (-)baclofen	16.00 ± 0.40
100 mM KCl + 5 X 10^{-6} M (-)baclofen	13.43 ± 1.40[a]
100 mM KCl + 10^{-5} M (-)baclofen	11.82 ± 1.20[b]
100 mM KCl + 5 X 10^{-5} M (-)baclofen	10.50 ± 0.74[b]
100 mM KCl + 10^{-4} M (-)baclofen	9.93 ± 0.94[b]
100 mM KCl + 5 X 10^{-4} M (-)baclofen	9.25 ± 0.90[b]

The results are the mean ± S.D. of four experiments.
[a] $P < 0.02$; [b] $P < 0.001$, as compared to 100 mM KCl. Reproduced with persmission from (14).

However, coupling of $GABA_B$ receptors to adenylate cyclase has been demonstrated (36). This may represent one of the additional differences between pre- and postsynaptic $GABA_B$ receptors. Furthermore, a recent study has shown that GABA and baclofen inhibited both the basal and forskolin stimulated adenylate cyclase activity, and this inhibitory effect was prevented by pertussis toxin (10). These results indicate coupling of $GABA_B$ receptors to both adenylate cyclase and G-proteins. Since we are measuring the end result of Ca^{2+}-influx followed by ^{86}Rb-efflux, it is feasible that the protein kinases could affect at different stages of the Ca^{2+}-activated ^{86}Rb-efflux. Thus, it is feasible that the effect of forskolin on protein kinase-A activation could be due to its ability to block Ca^{2+}-activated K^+-channels at a stage subsequent to Ca^{2+}-influx. Nonetheless, $GABA_B$ receptors are coupled to adenylate cyclase (28,35) and direct involvement of this system cannot be ruled out. However, it is worthwhile to note that nicotinic acetylcholine receptor can be phosphorylated by three different kinases, viz protein kinase-A, protein kinase-C, and tyrosine kinase. Finally, since there are apparently differences between pre- and postsynaptic $GABA_B$ receptors, we have suggested that presynaptic receptors be termed $GABA_{B1}$ and postsynaptic $GABA_{B2}$ (33).

TABLE 5. Effect of phorbol ester on the inhibition of ^{86}Rb-efflux by (-)baclofen in spinal cord neurons

Treatment	% ^{86}Rb-Efflux (Mean ± S.D.)	
	Without Phorbol Ester	With Phorbol Ester (10 µM)
5 mM KCl	5.25 ± 0.20	5.66 ± 0.50
100 mM KCl	15.26 ± 0.71	16.19 ± 2.12
100 mM KCl + 10^{-4} M (-)baclofen	11.07 ± 0.42[a]	15.37 ± 1.18

Coverslips were treated with or without phorbol ester (10 µM) for 20 min before starting the efflux studies, as described in "Methods." The results are mean ± S.D. of four experiments.
[a]$P < 0.01$, as compared to 100 mM KCl. Reproduced with permission from (14).

ACKNOWLEDGEMENTS

This work was supported in part by NIH-NINCDS grants NS15339, NS24339, and NIAAA grant AA040090.

REFERENCES

1. Allan, A. M. and Harris, A. R. (1988): Life Sci., 39:2005-2015.
2. Andrade, R., Malenka, K. C. and Nicoll, R. A. (1986): Science, 234:1261-1265.

3. Bartschat, D. R. and Blaustein, M. P. (1985): J. Physiol. (Lond.), 361:441-457.
4. Biggio, G. and Costa, E., editors (1988): Chloride Channels and Their Modulation by Neurotransmitters and Drugs. Raven Press, New York.
5. Bowery, N. G., Price, G. W., Hudson, A. L., Hill, D. R., Wilkin, G. P. and Turball, M. J. (1984): Neuropharmacol., 23:219-231.
6. Celentano, J. J., Gibbs, T. T. and Farb, D. H. (1988): Brain Res., 455:377-388.
7. Chan, C. Y. and Farb, D. H. (1985): J. Neurosci., 9:2365-2373.
8. Davidoff, R. A. (1973): Arch. Neurol., 28:60-63.
9. Dolphin, A. C. and Scott, R. H. (1987): J. Physiol. (Lond.), 386:1-17.
10. Dutar, P. and Nicoll, R. A. (1988): Neuron., 1:585-591.
11. Frye, G. D. and Breese, G. R. (1982): J. Pharmacol. Exp. Ther., 223:750-756.
12. Holz, G. G., Rane, S. G. and Dunlap, K. (1986): Nature, 319:670-672.
13. Jakobs, H., Bauer, S. and Watanabe, Y. (1985): Eur. J. Biochem., 151:425-430.
14. Kamatchi, G. L. and Ticku, M. K. (1989): Brain Res., In press.
15. Kerr, D. I. B., Ong, J., Prager, R. H., Gynther, B. D. and Curtis, D. R. (1987): Brain Res., 405:150-154.
16. Lehoullier, P. F. and Ticku, M. K. (1989): Brain Res., 487:205-214.
17. Liljequist, S. and Engel, J. (1982): Psychopharmacology, 78:71-75.
18. Lima-Landman, M. T. R. and Albaquerque, E. X. (1989): FEBS Lett., 247:61-67.
19. Lovinger, D. M., White, G. and Weight, F. F. (1989): Science, 243:1721-1725.
20. Madison, D. V. and Nicoll, R. A. (1986): J. Physiol., 372:245-252.
21. Mancillas, J. R., Siggins, G. R. and Bloom, F. E. (1986): Science, 231:161-164.
22. Mehta, A. K. and Ticku, M. K. (1987): J. Neurochem., 49:1491-1497.
23. Mehta, A. K. and Ticku, M. K. (1988): J. Pharmacol. Exp. Ther., 246:558-564.
24. Mehta, A. K. and Ticku, M. K. (1988): Brain Res., 454:156-163.
25. Mehta, A. K. and Ticku, M. K. (1989): J. Pharmacol. Exp. Ther., 249:418-423.
26. Nestoros, J. N. (1980): Science, 209:708-710.
27. Nishio, M. and Narahashi, T. (1988): Soc. Neurosci. Abst., 14:642.

28. Nishikawa, M. and Kuriyama, K. (1989): Neurochem. Int., 14:85-90.
29. Olsen, R. W. (1981): J. Neurochem., 37:1-13.
30. Polc, P., Mohler, H. and Haefely, W. (1974): Naunyn-Schmiedebergs Arch. Pharmac., 284:319-337.
31. Pritchett, D. B., Sontheimer, H., Shivers, B. D., Ymer, S., Kettenmann, H., Schofield, P. R. and Seeburg, P. H. (1989): Nature, 338:582-585.
32. Suzdak, P., Glowa, J. R., Crawley, J. N., Schwartz, R. D., Skolnick, P. and Paul, S. M. (1986): Science, 234:1243-1247.
33. Ticku, M. K. and Delgado, A. (1989): Life Sci., 44:1271-1276.
34. Ticku, M. K. and Kulkarni, S. K. (1988): Pharmacol. Biochem. Behav., 30:501-510.
35. Ticku, M. K. and Maksay, G. (1983): Life Sci., 33:2363-2375.
36. Wojcik, W. J. and Neff, N. H. (1984): Mol. Pharmacol., 25:24-28.

GABA and Benzodiazepine Receptor Subtypes,
edited by Giovanni Biggio and Erminio Costa.
Raven Press, New York © 1990.

CHRONIC ADMINISTRATION OF NEGATIVE MODULATORS PRODUCES CHEMICAL KINDLING AND GABA$_A$ RECEPTOR DOWN-REGULATION

M.G. Corda, O. Giorgi, M. Orlandi, B. Longoni
and G. Biggio

Department of Experimental Biology,
Chair of Pharmacology,
University of Cagliari, ITALY

A number of convulsant and anticonvulsant agents modify neuronal excitability by altering the GABA-gated chloride current through the neuronal membrane. Biochemical studies indicate that these effects are mediated by a set of multiple recognition sites located in the GABA$_A$ receptor complex. The availability of two biochemical tecniques, the uptake of $^{36}Cl^-$ and the binding of ^{35}S-t-butylbicyclophosphorothionate (^{35}S-TBPS) has allowed a detailed examination of the pharmacological regulation of the GABA-gated chloride channels (21, 45). "In vitro" studies have shown that the GABA-gated $^{36}Cl^-$ uptake is enhanced by positive modulators such as barbiturates and benzodiazepines, whereas it is reduced by negative modulators such as ß-carboline derivatives and chloride channel blockers (1, 33, 35, 42, 43, 51). Similarly, the binding of ^{35}S-TBPS to brain membranes is modulated by psychoactive drugs with a site of action on the GABA$_A$ receptor complex (6, 7, 17, 44, 45, 49).
It is well known that the repeated administration of positive modulators of GABAergic transmission produces tolerance to the effects of these drugs in experimental animals and in humans (20). This long-term pharmacological effect is associated with neurochemical alterations in the GABAergic system, as determined in a variety of animal models and tissue culture systems (see Miller et al., this volume). In contrast, the re-

peated administration of different GABA function inhibitors causes behavioral sensitization which results
in chemical kindling (10, 15, 24, 27, 31, 36, 37, 48).
This chapter will describe the studies carried out in
our laboratory over the last years to characterize the
behavioral and neurochemical consequences produced in
rats by the chronic treatment with negative modulators
acting at different sites of the GABA$_A$ receptor
complex.

KINDLING WITH FG 7142 AND THE GABA$_A$ RECEPTOR COMPLEX

FG 7142 (ß-carboline-3-carboxylic acid-methyl ami-
de) is a ß-carboline derivative which binds to benzodiazepine recognition sites and produces effects opposite to those of benzodiazepines (4). Thus, FG 7142
induces anxiety in animal models and in humans, enhances vigilance and is proconvulsant (8, 16, 34, 47).
Moreover, FG 7142 has a negative modulatory action on
central GABAergic transmission "in vitro", as indicated by its ability to reduce the binding of ^{3}H-GABA
and to increase the binding of ^{35}S-TBPS to neuronal
membranes (2, 6). The repeated administration of FG
7142 to rodents results in sensitization to its convulsant properties, so that the compound from proconvulsant becomes a full convulsant after several
injections. In rats, sensitization can be induced by a
variety of schedules of drug administration (i.e. twice a day, every day or three times a week injections
for a total of 20-30 injections) and is prevented by
the concurrent administration of the benzodiazepine
receptor antagonist flumazenil (3, 10, 12, 14).
Interestingly, chemical kindling produced by FG 7142
resembles electrical kindling in that both phenomena
are long-lasting. In rats, we observed the persistence
of kindling up to two months after the cessation of
the chronic treatment and an even longer duration of
sensitization to FG 7142 has been found by Little et
al. in mice (26).
Rats kindled with FG 7142 show an altered responsiveness to other benzodiazepine recognition site ligands.
Thus, proconvulsant agents such as Ro 15-4513 and ßCCE
produce full convulsions, whereas the behavioral effects of diazepam are reduced in rats kindled with FG
7142 (11, 12). In addition, kindled rats show an enhanced responsiveness to convulsions produced by isoniazid (10), a specific inhibitor of the GABA
synthesis. All these results, in agreement with data
from other laboratories showing a reduction in the efficacy of GABA mimetic drugs in FG 7142-kindled rats
(26, 29), may indicate a subsensitivity of the GABAergic system in the brain of these animals. To test this

possibility we measured a number of biochemical parameters of the GABAergic function in brain. The binding
parameters of ^{3}H-Flunitrazepam and ^{3}H-ßCCE are not modified in brain membranes from rats kindled with FG
7142. In contrast, the density of low affinity GABA
receptors is reduced in the cerebral cortex of kindled
rats sacrificed five days after the last drug administration (10). This effect is paralleled by a reduction in the stimulation produced by GABA on ^{36}Cl$^-$ uptake (12, 14). These findings are in agreement with
our previous report on the reduction of ^{3}H-GABA binding in the cerebral cortex of rats repeatedly injected with ßCCE (3, 5) and with data from other laboratories showing a reduction in the stimulatory effect
of GABA on benzodiazepine binding and on ^{36}Cl$^-$ uptake
in the brain of mice kindled with FG 7142 (25, 26).
Considered together, the above results support the
view that the long-lasting chemical kindling produced
by repeated exposure to FG 7142 may be associated to a
reduction in the function of the GABA$_A$/receptor
complex.

CHRONIC TREATMENT WITH PENTYLENETETRAZOL AND KINDLING

To further evaluate the behavioural and neurochemical effects produced by chronic administration of negative modulators of GABAergic function, in subsequent
experiments we used pentylenetetrazol (PTZ). This compound is a C.N.S. stimulant widely used in the screening of anxiolytic and anticonvulsant agents. Biochemical and electrophysiological studies indicate that
its pharmacological effects are due to a selective
blockade of the GABA-coupled chloride ionophore (30,
39, 46). Interestingly, PTZ, like FG 7142, has been
reported to produce chemical kindling in rats and mice
upon repeated administration (15, 24, 31, 37). Therefore we considered of interest to further characterize
PTZ-kindling in rats and to evaluate whether this effect is associated with modifications of the GABA$_A$ receptor complex in brain. The repeated administration
of subconvulsant doses of PTZ (30 mg/kg i.p., three
times a week) produces an increased susceptibility to
the drug whithin few weeks. In fact, starting from the
second week of treatment the percent of animals showing seizures increases until 80-90% of them are sen-
sitized by the end of the chronic treatment (10th
week) (Fig. 1). This PTZ-kindling persists for a long
time after drug discontinuation, since kindled rats
show convulsions when challenged with PTZ up to 8
months after the last drug administration (Table 1).
In contrast, convulsions are not observed in saline-
treated rats challenged with PTZ or, viceversa, in PTZ-

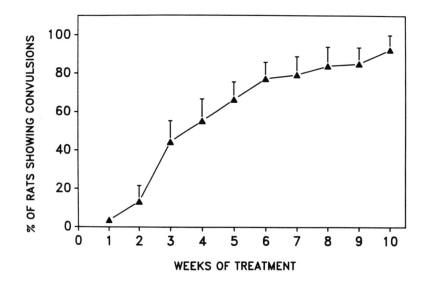

FIG. 1 <u>Sensitization to convulsions during chronic treatment with pentylenetetrazol (PTZ).</u>
PTZ (30 mg/kg, i.p.) was injected 3 times a week for 10 weeks. Rats were observed for 60 min after the injection and the number of animals displaying seizures was recorded. Results are expressed as percentages (mean $\pm$ S.E.M.) of convulsing rats. Data were obtained from 3 experiments (15 rats per experiment).

TABLE 1. EFFECT OF A CHALLENGE WITH PENTYLENETETRAZOL (PTZ) IN RATS REPEATEDLY INJECTED WITH SALINE OR PTZ

CHRONIC TREATMENT	CHALLENGE	N. OF ANIMALS SHOWING CONVULSIONS
Saline	Saline	0/5
Saline	PTZ	0/5
PTZ	Saline	0/6
PTZ	PTZ	5/6*

Rats were challenged with PTZ (20 mg/kg, i.p.) 8 months after the completion of the chronic treatment. *$p < 0.05$ vs the saline-PTZ group (Fisher's exact probability test).

kindled rats challenged with saline (Table 1). Therefore, this schedule of PTZ administration most probably produces permanent changes in the susceptibility to the drug.

In subsequent experiments we evaluated whether there is a cross sensitization between PTZ and other negative modulators of GABAergic transmission. Rats were challenged with the benzodiazepine receptor ligands FG 7142 (20 mg/kg i.p.), ßCCE (10 mg/kg i.v.) and Ro 15-4513 (10 mg/kg i.p.), 5 days after the last PTZ administration. In agreement with their pharmacological profile, the compounds are not convulsant in rats repeatedly injected with saline, whereas they produce full convulsions in 80% to 100% of rats kindled with PTZ (Table 2).

TABLE 2. EFFECT OF DIFFERENT BENZODIAZEPINE RECEPTOR LIGANDS IN RATS KINDLED WITH PTZ

CHALLENGE	N. OF ANIMALS SHOWING CONVULSIONS	
	SALINE	PTZ
FG 7142	0/5	5/5*
ßCCE	0/6	5/6*
Ro 15-4513	0/5	4/5*

Rats were challenged with FG 7142 (20 mg/kg, i.p.), ßCCE (10 mg/kg, i.v.) or Ro 15-4513 (10 mg/kg, i.p.) 5 days after the last PTZ administration. *p < 0.05 compared to the respective saline group (Fisher's exact probability test).

TABLE 3. INCREASED SUSCEPTIBILITY TO CONVULSIONS INDUCED BY ISONIAZID IN RATS KINDLED WITH PTZ

CHRONIC TREATMENT	N. OF RATS AFFECTED		
	CLONUS	TONUS	DEATH
Saline	9/10	3/10	1/10
PTZ	10/10	8/10*	6/10*

Rats were challenged with isoniazid (300 mg/kg, s.c.) five days after the completion of the chronic treatment and were observed for 2 hours after isoniazid injection. *p < 0.05 vs the respective saline group (Fisher's exact probability test).

Finally, we evaluated the susceptibility to convulsions induced by isoniazid in rats kindled with PTZ. As mentioned above, the convulsive effect of isoniazid is due to the blockade of the enzyme which synthetizes GABA (glutamic acid decarboxylase) that leads to a decreased availability of this inhibitory neurotransmitter at the synaptic level (22). Isoniazid was administered subcutaneously at the dose of 300 mg/kg to saline or PTZ-treated rats, five days after the completion of the chronic treatment. No differences in the percentage of rats showing myoclonic seizures were observed between the two experimental groups, whereas there was a significant increase in the number of rats showing prolonged periods of tonic hindlimb extensions followed by death in the PTZ group (Table 3).

CHRONIC TREATMENT WITH PENTYLENETETRAZOL AND THE GABA_A RECEPTOR COMPLEX

Previous studies indicate that PTZ blocks GABA-mediated inhibitory transmission through an action on the convulsant binding site on the GABA_A receptor com-

TABLE 4. EFFECT OF ACUTE AND CHRONIC TREATMENT WITH PTZ ON ^{35}S-TBPS BINDING TO CEREBRAL CORTEX MEMBRANES

TREATMENT	SPECIFIC ^{35}S-TBPS BINDING	
	Bmax (pmol/mg prot)	K_D (nM)
ACUTE		
Saline	2.11 ± 0.16	53 ± 4
PTZ 25 mg	2.05 ± 0.14	61 ± 2
PTZ 50 mg	1.88 ± 0.11	58 ± 4
PTZ 75 mg	1.91 ± 0.15	56 ± 3
CHRONIC		
Saline	2.25 ± 0.10	58 ± 5
PTZ	1.68 ± 0.15*	55 ± 4

Rats were sacrificed 20 min and 3 days after acute and chronic PTZ administration, respectively. ^{35}S-TBPS binding was measured as previously described (14) using 2-320 nM of ^{35}S-TBPS. Each value is the mean ± S.E.M. of 3 separate experiments for acute and 8 experiments for chronic PTZ, each run in triplicate. *p < 0.01 vs the respective saline group (Student's t-test).

plex (39, 46). Accordingly, the "in vitro" addition of
PTZ to cerebral cortex membrane preparations displaces
the specific binding of ^{35}S-TBPS in a concentration-
dependent manner, with an IC_{50} value of 860 ± 60 μM (13).
It is noteworthy that this IC_{50} value is in the range
of concentrations achieved in brain after the "in
vivo" administration of a convulsant dose (52). The
Scatchard analysis of saturation binding data shows
that 800 μM PTZ causes a two-fold increase of the apparent dissociation constant without altering the Bmax
value, indicating that PTZ is a competitive inhibitor
of ^{35}S-TBPS binding (13).
In a preliminary set of experiments we evaluated the
effect of the acute administration of PTZ on ^{35}S-TBPS
binding. To this aim, rats were injected intraperitoneally with different doses of PTZ (25-75 mg/kg) and
were sacrificed 20 min thereafter; ^{35}S-TBPS binding
was measured the same day in fresh cerebral cortex

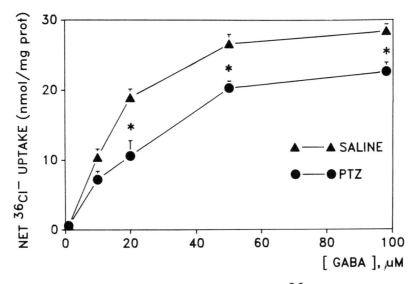

FIG. 2   Decrease of GABA-stimulated ^{36}Cl$^-$ uptake in
the cerebral cortex of rats chronically trea-
ted with PTZ.
Rats were sacrificed 3 days after the last PTZ
administration. ^{36}Cl$^-$ uptake was assayed as
previously described (14) in the absence or
presence of GABA (10-100 μM) using pooled tissue from 2 rats. Results are the mean $\pm$ S.E.M.
from 4 separate experiments run in quintupli-
cate. Basal ^{36}Cl$^-$ uptake (nmol ^{36}Cl$^-$/mg prot)
in the two experimental groups was as follows:
saline 11.1 $\pm$ 0.7; PTZ 13.1 $\pm$ 1.2.
*p < 0.02 vs the respective saline group.

membrane preparations. Neither treatment with PTZ modifies the specific binding of ^{35}S-TBPS to different brain areas, indicating that the compound, due to its low affinity for ^{35}S-TBPS binding sites, is rapidly removed during membrane preparation (Table 4).
On the other hand, the repeated administration of PTZ (30 mg/kg i.p., 3 times a week for 10 weeks) decreases by 26% the density of ^{35}S-TBPS binding sites in the cerebral cortex, without altering the dissociation constant (Table 4). This effect is observed at 3 and 6 days after the last PTZ administration. To study whether or not the decrease in ^{35}S-TBPS binding is associated with modifications of chloride channel function, we measured the uptake of ^{36}Cl$^-$ into membrane vesicles from the cerebral cortex of saline and PTZ-treated rats. As indicated in Fig. 2, the stimulation of ^{36}Cl$^-$ uptake produced by GABA is smaller in the PTZ group as compared to controls, at all the concentrations of GABA used (10 - 100 μM), whereas no significant differences in the basal uptake between the two experimental groups are observed.

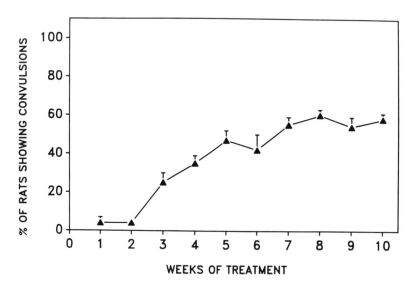

FIG. 3   <u>Sensitization to convulsions during chronic treatment with picrotoxin</u>
Picrotoxin (2 mg/kg i.p.) was injected 3 times a week for 10 weeks. Rats were observed for 1 hour after each injection and the number of animals displaying seizures was recorded. Results are expressed as percentages (mean $\pm$ S.E.M.) of convulsing rats. Data were obtained from 3 experiments (10 rats per experiment).

CHRONIC ADMINISTRATION OF PICROTOXIN PRODUCES KINDLING AND DECREASES ^{35}S-TBPS BINDING

The results shown above are consistent with the hypothesis that the repeated administration of PTZ reduces the activity of the GABA-coupled chloride channel, an effect that may be associated to the chemical kindling produced by this drug. To verify this hypothesis further, rats were treated chronically with picrotoxin and their susceptibility to convulsions as well as the binding of ^{35}S-TBPS to cerebral cortex membranes was evaluated. Picrotoxin, a mixture of picrotoxinin and picrotoxin, is a selective blocker of the GABA-gated chloride channel that produces convulsions and experimental anxiety in rats (9, 34, 45). Accordingly, the "in vitro" addition of picrotoxin inhibits the binding of ^{35}S-TBPS in a concentration-dependent manner with an IC_{50} value of 300 nM. The inhibition of ^{35}S-TBPS binding by picrotoxin is competive, as indicated by the Scatchard plot analysis of saturation binding data. Thus, picrotoxin does not change the Bmax value, but causes a two-fold increase in the apparent dissociation constant of ^{35}S-TBPS binding (Control, Bmax 2.2 $\pm$ 0.28 pmol/mg prot, K_D 61 $\pm$ 5 nM; picrotoxin, Bmax 2.0 $\pm$ 0.15 pmol/mg prot, K_D 131 $\pm$ 15* nM. *p < 0.005, n = 4).
To evaluate the behavioral effects of chronic picrotoxin administration, rats were injected intraperitoneally with 2 mg/kg of picrotoxin three times a week and were observed for 1 hour after each drug administration. As indicated in Fig. 3, this treatment produces a consistent degree of sensitization. In fact, in

TABLE 5. EFFECT OF CHRONIC TREATMENT WITH PICROTOXIN ON ^{35}S-TBPS BINDING TO CEREBRAL CORTEX MEMBRANES

TREATMENT	SPECIFIC ^{35}S-TBPS BINDING	
	Bmax (pmol/mg prot)	K_D (nM)
Saline	2.15 $\pm$ 0.12	54 $\pm$ 4
Picrotoxin	1.62 $\pm$ 0.11*	61 $\pm$ 7

Rats were sacrificed 3 days after the last drug administration. ^{35}S-TBPS binding was measured as described in Table 4. Each value is the mean $\pm$ S.E.M. of 7 experiments, each run in triplicate. *p < 0.01 vs saline.

the first two weeks of treatment there are no signs of convulsive activity, whereas starting from the third week an increasing number of animals show convulsions, until approximately 50% of them are affected by the 6th week of treatment. No further increase in sensitization is observed during the following weeks, even after 10 weeks of treatment (Fig. 3). The binding of ^{35}S-TBPS was measured three days after the completion of the chronic treatment only in those rats which developed sensitization to picrotoxin. In agreement with the results obtained with PTZ, there is a significant decrease in the density of ^{35}S-TBPS binding sites in the cerebral cortex of rats kindled with picrotoxin as compared to saline-treated rats (Table 5).

CONCLUSIONS

The term kindling refers to a phenomenon in which the repeated administration of a subconvulsive electrical stimulus results in progressive intensification of seizure activity. This phenomenon, originally described by Goddard in 1967 (18), was also described after the repeated administration of a variety of drugs (31, 37, 38). Our study, in agreement with those reports, indicates that chemical kindling can be induced by different negative modulators of GABAergic transmission, such as FG 7142, pentylenetetrazol and picrotoxin. Like electrical kindling, the chemical kindling produced by these agents is rather long-lasting, indicating that it induces a permanent decrease in seizure threshold in brain.
There is extensive evidence suggesting that alterations in GABAergic neurotransmission plays an important role in convulsive disorders (23, 28, 40, 41). Thus, a variety of factors which decrease GABAergic function produce seizures, whereas factors which enhance GABAergic function reduce seizure susceptibility (19, 22, 32, 44). Our study is consistent with the hypothesis that kindling produced by FG 7142, pentylenetetrazol and picrotoxin may be associated with deficits in GABAergic neurotransmission. Accordingly, rats kindled with these agents show an enhanced susceptibility to pharmacological treatments that reduce GABAergic activity in brain. Moreover, a decrease in GABAergic parameters (i.e. GABA receptors, ^{35}S-TBPS binding sites and GABA-gated chloride flux) is present in the cerebral cortex of rats kindled with FG 7142, pentylenetetrazol or picrotoxin. The involvement of other neurotransmitter systems in the chemical kindling produced by GABA function inhibitors cannot be ruled out at present. In this context, it is noteworthy that MK-801, the non-competitive antagonist of N-methyl-D-as-

partate receptors (50), has been recently found to prevent the development of kindling produced by FG 7142 (48). Work is now in progress to examine the possible contribution of excitatory aminoacids to the chemical kindling produced by negative modulators of GABAergic neurotransmission.

REFERENCES

1. Allan A.M. and Harris R.A. (1986): Mol. Pharmacol., 29: 497-505.

2. Biggio G., Concas A., Serra M., Salis M., Corda M.G., Nurchi V., Crisponi C. and Gessa G.L. (1984): Brain Res., 305: 13-18.

3. Biggio G., Giorgi O., Concas A. and Corda M.G. (1989): In: Allosteric Modulation of Amino Acid Receptors: Therapeutic Implications, edited by E.A. Barnard and E. Costa, pp. 71-89, Raven Press, New York.

4. Braestrup C., Honore' T., Nielsen M., Petersen E.N. and Jensen L.H. (1984): Biochem. Pharmacol., 33: 859-862.

5. Concas A., Salis M., Serra M., Corda M.G. and Biggio G. (1983): Eur. J. Pharmacol., 89: 179-181.

6. Concas A., Serra M., Atsoggiu T. and Biggio G. (1988): J. Neurochem., 51: 1868-1876.

7. Concas A., Serra M., Corda M.G. and Biggio G. (1988): In: Chloride Channels and Their Modulation by Neurotransmitters and Drugs, edited by G. Biggio and E. Costa, pp. 227-246, Raven Press, New York.

8. Corda M.G., Blaker W.D., Mendelson W.B., Guidotti A. and Costa E. (1983): Proc. Natl. Acad. Sci. USA, 80: 2072-2076.

9. Corda M.G. and Biggio G. (1986): Neuropharmacol., 25: 521-524.

10. Corda M.G., Giorgi O. and Biggio G. (1986): Brain Res., 384: 60-67.

11. Corda M.G., Giorgi O., Longoni B. and Biggio G. (1988): Neurosci. Lett., 86: 219-224.

12. Corda M.G., Giorgi O., Longoni B., Fernandez A.

and Biggio G.: In: Chloride Channels and their Modulation by Neurotransmitters and Drugs edited by G. Biggio and E. Costa, pp. 293-306. Raven Press, New York.

13. Corda M.G., Giorgi O., Longoni B., Orlandi M. and Biggio G. (1990): J. Neurochem. (in press).

14. Corda M.G., Longoni B., Giorgi O., Fernandez A. and Biggio G. (1988): Neurosci. Res. Comm., 3: 167-174.

15. Diehl R.G., Smialowski A. and Gotwo T. (1984): Epilepsia, 25: 506-510.

16. Dorow R., Horowski R., Paschelke G., Amin M. and Braestrup C. (1983) Lancet, 2: 98-99.

17. Gee K.W., Lawrence L.J. and Yamamura H.I. (1986): Mol. Pharmacol., 30: 218-225.

18. Goddard G.V. (1967): Nature, 214: 1020-1021.

19. Haefely W.E. (1980): Brain Res. Bull., 5 (Suppl. 2): 873-878.

20. Haigh J.R.M. and Feely M. (1988): TIPS, 9: 361-366.

21. Harris R.A. and Allan A.M. (1985): Science, 228: 1108-1110.

22. Horton R.W. (1980): Brain Res. Bull., 5 (Suppl. 2): 605-608.

23. Houser C.R., Harris A.B. and Vaughn J.E. (1986): Brain Res., 383: 129-145.

24. Karler R., Murphy V., Calder L.D. and Turkanis S.A. (1989): Neuropharmacol., 28: 775-780.

25. Lewin E., Peris J., Bleck V., Zahniser N.R. and Harris R.A. (1989): Eur. J. Pharmacol., 160: 101-106.

26. Little H.J., Nutt D.J. and Taylor S.C. (1987): J. Psychopharmacol., 1: 35-46.

27. Little H.J., Nutt D.J. and Taylor S.C. (1984): Br. J. Pharmac., 83: 951-958.

28. Lloyd K.G., Munari C., Bossi L. and Morselli P.L.

(1984): In: Neurotransmitters, Seizures and Epilepsy II edited by R.G. Fariello, P.L. Morselli, K.G. Lloyd L.F. Quesney, J. Engel, pp. 285-293. Raven Press, New York.

29. Loscher W. and Stephens D.N. (1988): Epilepsy Res., 2: 253-259.

30. MacDonald R.L. and Barker J.L. (1977) Nature, 267: 720-721.

31. Mason C.R. and Cooper R.M. (1972): Epilepsia, 13: 663-674.

32. Matthews W.D. and McCafferty (1979): Neuropharmacol., 18: 885-889.

33. Morrow A.L. and Paul S.M. (1988) J. Neurochem., 50: 302-306.

34. Nutt D.J., Cowen P.J. and Green A.R. (1980): Neuropharmacol., 19: 1017-1023.

35. Obata T. and Yamamura H.I. (1986): Biochem. Biophys. Res. Comm., 141: 1-6.

36. Petersen E.N. and Jensen L.H. (1987): Eur. J. Pharmacol., 133: 309-317.

37. Pinel J.P.J. and Cheung K.F. (1977): Pharm. Biochem. & Behav., 6: 599-600.

38. Post R.M. (1980): Life Sci., 26: 1275-1282.

39. Ramanjaneyulu R. and Ticku M.J. (1984) Eur. J. Pharmacol., 98: 337-345.

40. Ribak C.E., Harris A.B., Vaughn J.E. and Roberts E. (1979) Science, 205: 211-214.

41. Ross S.M. and Craig C.R. (1981): J. Neurosci., 1: 1388-1396.

42. Schwartz R.D., Jackson J.A., Weigert D., Skolnick P. and Paul S.M. (1985): J. Neurosci., 5: 2963-2970.

43. Serra M., Concas A., Atsoggiu T. and Biggio G. (1988): Neurosci. Res. Comm., 4: 41-50.

44. Serra M., Sanna E. and Biggio G. (1989): Eur. J. Pharmacol., 164: 385-388.

45. Squires R.F., Casida J.E., Richardson M. and Saederup E. (1983): Mol. Pharmacol., 23: 326-336.

46. Squires R.F., Saederup E., Crawley J.N., Skolnick P. and Paul S.M. (1984): Life Sci., 35: 1439-1444.

47. Stephens D.N. and Sarter M. (1988): In: Benzodiazepine Receptor Ligands: Memory and Information Processing, edited by I. Hindmarch and H. Ott., pp. 205-217. Springer, Berlin.

48. Stephens D.N. and Weidmann R. (1989): Brain Res., 492: 89-98.

49. Supavilai P. and Karobath M. (1984): J. Neurosci., 4: 1193-1200.

50. Wong E.H., Kemp J.A., Priestley T., Knight A.R., Woodruff G.N. and Iversen L.L. (1986): Proc. Natl. Acad. Sci. USA, 83: 7104-7108.

51. Wong E.H., Leeb-Lundberg L.M.F., Teichberg V.I. and Olsen R.W. (1983): Brain Res., 303: 267-275.

52. Yonekawa W.D., Kupferberg H.J. and Woodbury D.M. (1980): J. Pharmacol. Exp. Ther., 214: 589-593.

GABA and Benzodiazepine Receptor Subtypes,
edited by Giovanni Biggio and Erminio Costa.
Raven Press, New York © 1990.

CHRONIC BENZODIAZEPINE ADMINISTRATION:

EFFECTS *IN VIVO* AND *IN VITRO*

Lawrence G. Miller, David J. Greenblatt, Fred Lopez, Andrew Schatzki,
Jack Heller, Monica Lumpkin and Richard I. Shader

From the Division of Clinicial Pharmacology, Depts. of Psychiatry and
Pharmacology, Tufts Univ. School of Medicine and New England Medical Center,
Boston, MA 02111, USA

Benzodiazepines are in widespread use as anxiolytics, hypnotics, and anticonvulsants (15). Abundant neurochemical evidence indicates that benzodiazepines exert their effects in the central nervous system at a speific binding site on the GABAa receptor complex (16). Although clinical use of benzodiazepines generally involves chronic dosage, most neurochemical studies have evaluated acute effects of benzodiazepines. This review will consider studies of chronic benzodiazepine administration, in particular methodologic issues, and discuss the use of a tissue culture model to examine neurochemical effects of benzodiazepine administration. Several recent reports have addressed behavioral effects of chronic benzodiazepine administration; behavioral effects will be considered here only briefly (33,50).

Chronic administration of benzodiazepines has been reported to produce tolerance to the effects of these drugs in humans and animals (9,10,14,20,49), but the mechanism of benzodiazepine tolerance remains uncertain. Most pharmacokinetic studies of chronic dosage in animals and humans found little change in steady-state plasma concentrations after prolonged dosage (14,15,17). Although little evidence is available concerning effects of chronic administration on uptake of benzodiazepines from plasma to brain, several recent studies in mice indicate no change in brain concentrations during two weeks of drug administration by continuous infusion (26,28,29). Thus, it is unlikely that pharmacokinetic alterations can account for the attenuation of behavioral effects observed during chronic drug administration.

ANIMAL STUDIES: BENZODIAZEPINE AGONISTS

Chronic Agonist Administration

Soon after the description of the benzodiazepine binding site in brain, a number of investigators assessed effects of chronic benzodiazepine agonist administration on benzodiazepine receptor binding. Results of these initial studies were conflicting. Two studies (Mohler et al. (32); Braestrup et al. (2)) reported no change in binding, while several studies (Chiu and Rosenberg (3); Rosenberg and Chiu (37,38)) found decreases in binding, and one study indicated an increase in binding (DiStefano et al. (7)). These discrepancies may be due in part to differences in drugs and dosage schedules. Of studies indicating no change, Mohler et al. (32) used diazepam, 3 mg/kg i.p. daily for 3 weeks and Braestrup et al. (2) used diazepam, 90 mg/kg p.o daily for 8 weeks. Chiu and Rosenberg (3) used flurazepam, 100-150 mg/kg for 1 to 4 weeks, while DiStefano et al. (7) used diazepam 170 mg/kg p.o. daily for 5 weeks. All investigators used rats, and in no case were plasma or brain concentrations determined. Thus, even among investigators using diazepam, there was a nearly 60-fold range in administered dose, and differences in route of administration provde further variability among studies. In addition, diazepam and flurazepam differ markedly in metabolism, brain uptake, and receptor occupancy, although both have long-half-life metabolites in rodents and humans. Without drug analyses, it is difficult to ensure chronic brain concentrations or to identify the metabolite likely to account for alterations. Similarly, variability in length of dosage make comparisons difficult. Finally, the interval between final dose and receptor analysis adds possible variability. In most studies, tissue was removed 14-28 hours after the final dose, so that either a gradual onset or rapidly decaying effect might be missed. In a review of some of these early studies, Overstreet and Yamamura (34) found no clear basis for modulation of benzodiazepine binding during chronic drug administration.

Subsequent studies also yielded varying results, and comparisons among studies remained difficult. Abracchio et al. (1) reported a decrease in benzodiazepine receptor number in several brain regions of rats treated for 3 weeks with chlordiazepoxide. In contrast, Medina et al. (24) found little change in binding in cortex of rats treated with diazepam p.o. for 2 weeks, and Reeves and Schweizer (35) reported an increase in binding in rats receiving diazepam twice daily. Several studies indicated the specificity of binding effects for individual drugs. Scharf and Feil (41) reported an increase in receptor number after treatment for one week with lorazepam and clonazepam, while Crawley et al. (6) found a decrease in forebrain binding after 3 weeks of increasing doses of clonazepam but not chlordiazepoxide. As in earlier studies, drug concentrations were not determined, and variations in dosage schedule and the interval between dosage and binding analysis render comparisons uncertain.

More recently, several investigators have addressed both benzodiazepine binding and GABAa receptor function after chronic benzodiazepine agonist administration, as well as effects of chronic benzodiazepine antagonist and inverse agonist treatment. In a series of studies, Gallager and colleagues (11-13,18,23) used chronic infusion of diazepam by implanted capsules to assess binding at several sites on the GABAa receptor, as well as electrophysiologic indices of GABA sensitivity and neurochemical determinations of chloride flux. No changes in binding of an agonist, antagonist, and inverse agonist were observed after three weeks of treatment, although GABA inhibition of inverse agonist binding was altered. No change in binding at the putative chloride channel site labeled by [^{35}S]TBPS was observed. Electrophysiologic studies indicated decreases in the iontophoretic sensitivity to GABA in both the dorsal raphe nucleus and the substantia nigra pars reticulata. Finally, GABA-stimulated chloride uptake was decreased in diazepam-treated rats. Somewhat different results were reported by Chiu and Rosenberg and colleagues (39,48,51), using oral administration of diazepam or flurazepam in rats over 4 weeks. Decreases in benzodiazepine binding in cortex and hippocampus were observed, beginning approximately 1 week after drug administration. In chloride uptake studies, no changes were found in GABA-stimulated uptake, but benzodiazepine enhancement of GABA effects was reduced at 12 hours but not 48 hours after termination of drug administration.

We have recently performed a series of experiments examining the effects of chronic benzodiazepine administration on GABAa receptor binding and function (26,29). Using chronic infusion by implanted osmotic pumps, we demonstrated no change in plasma or brain drug concentrations for up to 2 weeks of administration using lorazepam (26) and alprazolam (29). In each instance, we found a decrease in benzodiazepine receptor binding apparently due to decreased receptor number in mice assessed during chronic adminstration. Binding was decreased in cortex and several other brain regions after 7 days of lorazepam and clonazepam, and 4 days of alprazolam. These results are similar to those reported for flurazepam by Tietz et al. (48). For both lorazepam and alprazolam, binding reverted rapidly to control levels, in each case by 24 hours after drug discontinuation, and in both cases increases in binding were observed 48 to 96 hours after drug discontinuation. No consistent changes were observed in chloride channel binding, as observed by Gallager and colleagues for chronic diazepam.

With regard to GABAa receptor function, we found decreases in GABA-dependent chloride uptake in mice chronically treated with lorazepam, alprazolam, or clonazepam. Uptake at low doses of the GABA analog muscimol was unchanged, but maximal uptake was substantially decreased in each case. The time course of changes in chloride uptake was similar to that observed for benzodiazepine binding. Results of chloride uptake studies are thus similar to those reported by Marley and Gallager (21) for chronic diazepam treatment, and parallel findings by Gallager and colleagues (13) based on electrophysiologic techniques. The data are in contrast to those of Yu et al. (51) based on chronic flurazepam administration.

Methodologic issues

Thus, despite a decade of study, data are conflicting concerning the neurochemical effects of chronic benzodiazepine agonist administration. Several methodologic issues can be identified in this literature. First, use of various benzodiazepines, and in particular benzodiazepines with active metabolites, limits comparability of studies. For example, diazepam is metabolized in rodents and humans to desmethyldiazepam, temazepam, and oxazepam, so it is unclear which compound affects GABAa characteristics. Similarly, flurazepam is metabolized to desalkylflurazepam and hydroxyethylflurazepam. Second, it is imperative to determine benzodiazepine concentrations in brain both to ensure adequate drug delivery and to allow comparisons among studies. Direct measurement of drug concentrations is preferable to indirect(e.g., radioreceptor) methods both for accuracy and in the case of multiple metabolites, for specificity. Third, the dosage interval and route of administration should be chosen to maintain significant drug concentrations in brain. This is especially true for drugs administered i.p. in rodents, since uptake and clearance are rapid. Under these conditions, benzodiazepines may be present in brain only transiently, even with multiple daily injections. It is uncertain whether such a pattern is an adequate model of chronic administration. Indeed, in clinical use, benzodiazepines are usually administered at intervals equal to or less than drug half-life (15). Thus, even with shorter-acting benzodiazepines(with the exception of triazolam) significant brain concentrations are maintained, and with longer-acting drugs such as diazepam or flurazepam virtually constant steady-state levels of metabolites are present. In sum, pharmacokinetic determinants require careful choice of drug and dosage interval and direct measurement of benzodiazepine concentrations in brain using specific analytical methods.

Timing of neurochemical analyses is also critical to ensure accurate results and to allow comparison among studies. Many investigators have assessed neurochemical parameters at an interval after the last dose or exposure to drug. Although this interval allows partial or complete clearance of drug, in turn avoiding interference with assays, the results may not accurately reflect changes due to chronic drug administration. As we and others have demonstrated (27,48), changes in benzodiazepine binding after chronic drug administration may resolve rapidly, and thus may be missed 24 hours after discontinuation. In addition, we have also demonstrated that opposite effects to those observed during chronic drug may be present as early as 48 hours after discontinuation (27). Thus, it is reasonable to perform neurochemical assays at steady-state drug concentrations. Comparison with vehicle-treated animals may not be possible due to presence of drug, but comparions can be made to acute or short-term drug administration.

ANIMAL STUDIES: BENZODIAZEPINE ANTAGONISTS AND INVERSE AGONISTS

Benzodiazepine Antagonists

Several studies have been performed involving chronic administration of benzodiazepine antagonists and inverse agonists. Soon after the identification of Ro15-1788(flumazenil) as a specific benzodiazepine antagonist, two investigators assessed neurochemical effects of chronic administration of this compound. Spirt et al. (45) reported no change in benzodiazepine binding in mice treated with flumazenil(50 mg/kg) i.p. three times per day for 3 days. In contrast, Medina et al. (25) found increases in binding in several brain regions in rats receiving 4 mg/kg p.o. in drinking water. As noted above, in the absence of brain concentrations, comparison of these studies is difficult due to marked differences in dosage schedules.

Recently, we examined effects of chronic flumazenil administration on GABAa receptor binding and function (28). Flumazenil concentrations were constant in brain up to 14 days at several administered doses. Benzodiazepine and TBPS binding were increased after 7 days, and GABA-dependent chloride uptake was also increased at this time point. These results are similar to binding data reported by Medina (25). The data suggest that the GABAa receptor complex shares with other neurotransmitter receptors the capacity to upregulate with chronic antagonist administration, in particular a benzodiazepine antagonist (19,40).

Benzodiazepine Inverse Agonists

Limited data are also available concerning the neurochemical effects of chronic FG 7142 administration. Corda et al. (4) reported that GABAa receptor density was decreased in cortex 5 days after FG 7142 discontinuation in rats. Subsequently, these authors found a decrease in GABA-dependent chloride uptake several days after FG 7142 administration (5). These results may be affected by the use of intermittent i.p. injections of FG 7142, which is rapidly cleared in rodents. In addition, as discussed above determinations several days after administration may be confounded by rapid changes in receptor binding and function after drug discontinuation. Studies in which drug concentrations are maintained and assays are performed during administration are necessary to confirm effects of chronic inverse agonists.

TISSUE CULTURE STUDIES

Chronic Agonist Administration

In an effort to avoid methodologic difficulties associated with animal studies, several investigators examined effects of chronic benzodiazepine agonist administration in tissue culture systems. These studies have relied on primary neuron cultures, since cell lines expressing the GABAa receptor have not been available. Studies have addressed effects on benzodiazepine binding and in some cases coupling to GABA, but not function of the GABAa receptor complex. Initial studies by Shibla et al. (44) reported no change in benzodiazepine binding in mouse-derived cultures treated for 3 weeks with diazepam, 1 uM. Similar results were reported by Farb et al. (8) in a chick system and by Maloteaux et al. (23) in rat-derived cultures. In contrast, Sher et al. (42) reported decreased binding in mouse spinal cord cultuers exposed to diazepam for 1 week. Electrophysiologic potentiation of GABA was also decreased after treatment. Subsequently, Sher and Machen (43) found similar decreases in binding in mouse-derived cortical cell cultures after exposure to clonazepam, 200 nM, for 14 days. Recently, Roca et al. (36) reported no change in benzodiazepine binding in chick cortical cultures after chronic flurazepam (10 uM), but a decrease in coupling of the benzodiazepine and GABA sites.

These conflicting results are analogous to those obtained in intact animals. Differences in species, culture conditions, drug exposure, and binding techniques make it difficult to compare studies. In addition, benzodiazepine binding alterations may not reflect changes in GABAa receptor function, as noted in animal studies. Thus, just as the introduction of chloride uptake techniques has markedly expanded studies in intact animal models, similar assessment of GABA-dependent chloride flux in drug-exposed culture systems is critical in determining chronic drug effects. Methods to assess chloride uptake in tissue culture have been reported by Thampy and Barnes (47), and we have recently modified these techniques for use in cultures chronically treated with clonazepam.

We used chick cerebral cortical neurons obtained from embryos incubated for 7-9 days, and subsequently cells are cultured for 10 days in serum-containing medium. These cultures yield nearly pure(>95%) populations of neurons with extensive network formation. The GABAa receptor in these cells appears to be very similar to the mammalian receptor (20), and we and others have characterized the dynamics of receptor binding during the culture period (46). Benzodiazepine, GABA, and TBPS receptors are present at the beginning of culture, and increase throughout the 10-day culture period. Subsequently, receptor numbers decrease rapidly, in part to due growth of non-neuronal cells. GABA-dependent chloride uptake can be assessed over a 10-second interval and corrected for cell number as determined by protein concentration.

In our initial studies (30), we assessed the effects of 1 uM clonazepam on muscimol-stimulated chloride uptake in neurons cultured for 10 days, and treated for the final 2 and 4 days, or the entire period of culture. After an acute (1 hour) exposure to this clonazepam concentration, uptake was increased at lower doses of muscimol(2-25 uM) but maximal uptake at 100 uM muscimol was unchanged. After treatment for 2 and 4 days, uptake across a range of muscimol concentrations was unchanged compared to vehicle-treated controls. However, after 10 days of drug exposure, uptake was decreased by 50-60% at all doses of muscimol evaluated. Treatment for 10 days with clonazepam, 0.1 uM, produced a smaller(30%) change, and a dose of 10 uM produced a greater(70-80%) decrement.

It is unlikely that these results are due to an alteration in chloride uptake characteristics or cell growth or survival. Uptake kinetics were unchanged in treated cells, and percentage of neuronal cells and total cellular protein were also unaffected. In addition, protein synthesis and degradation were not altered by chronic clonazepam treatment. To assess the mechanism for the decrease in chloride uptake, we determined benzodiazepine receptor binding in treated cells after dialysis to remove residual drug. Consistent with the results reported by Sher (42,43), we found a decrease in benzodiazepine receptor number after 10 days of clonazepam. These results suggest the possibility of a decrease in GABAa receptors associated with drug administration. In addition, we evaluated effects of concurrent administration of clonazepam, 0.1 uM, and Ro15-1788, 0.1 uM. In contrast to decreases in uptake observed with clonazepam alone, addition of Ro15-1788 returned uptake to control levels. These data support a specific effect of chronic clonazepam mediated by the benzodiazepine receptor, rather than a nonspecific effect on cell membranes or metabolism.

In summary, tissue culture systems allow evaluation of chronic benzodiazepine agonist administration in the absence of counfounding variables which may occur in intact animals. Prior data concerning benzodiazepine receptor binding is conflicting, indicating both decreases and no change in binding. We recently reported decreased GABA-dependent chloride uptake in cultures treated with chronic clonazepam. Additional studies may extend these findings to other benzodiazepines, as well as characterizing kinetics and specificity of this effect.

Chronic Antagonist and Inverse Agonist Administration

No prior studies have assessed benzodiazepine receptor binding or GABAa receptor function after chronic antagonist or inverse agonist exposure in tissue culture. Recently, we evaluated effects of chronic Ro15-1788 and FG 7142 administration on GABAa receptor function in cultured chick cortical neurons (31). Acute exposure(1 hour) to 1 uM Ro15-1788 had no effect on muscimol-stimulated chloride uptake. After 2 days of administration, chloride uptake was markedly increased at muscimol concentrations greater than 5 uM, and maximal uptake was increased by approximately 80%. Similar results were observed after 4 and 10 days of exposure. Ro15-1788, 0.1 uM, had no effect on chloride uptake after 10 days, , but a dose of 10 uM was significantly more potent than the 1 uM dose.

Acute administration(1 hour) of FG 7142 decreased chloride uptake at muscimol concentrations of 2-25 uM, but maximal uptake was not significantly affected. However, after 2 days, maximal chloride uptake was markedly increased(75-80%), and similar results were found after 4 and 10 days of drug exposure. FG 7142, 0.1 uM, had no effect on chloride uptake after 10 days, and results were similar with 1 uM and 10 uM doses.

With both chronic Ro15-1788 and FG 7142, no changes were observed in numbers of non-neuronal cells, total cellular protein, or protein synthesis and degradation. Thus, it is likely that increases in chloride uptake associated with chronic antagonist and inverse agonist administration are specific effects of benzodiazepines. These data illustrate the utility of tissue cultures systems in evaluating chronic benzodiazepine effects, but additional studies are necessary with these and other compounds to determine the effects of benzodiazepine antagonists and inverse agonists in detail.

SUMMARY

Chronic benzodiazepine administration is associated with neurochemical alterations in the GABAergic system, as determined in a variety of animal models and tissue culture systems. In animals, effects of chronic benzodiazepine agonists on receptor binding are uncertain, but several studies indicate a decrease in GABA-dependent chloride uptake. In contrast, limited data indicate that chloride uptake is increased after chronic antagonist administration, and results of inverse agonist administration are uncertain. Most animal studies are limited by lack of attention to drug choice and to pharmacokinetic variables, and by failure to determined delivered drug concentrations. More limited data in tissue culture systems are conflicting with regard to effects on benzodiazepine binding, but recent studies indicate that GABA-dependent chloride uptake may be decreased after chronic agonist exposure, and increased after chronic antagonist and inverse agonist administration. Data from these systems may complement results obtained in intact animals, and cultures may allow more detailed examination of the kinetics and specificity of drug effects.

References

1. Abbracchio MP, Balduini W, Coen E, Lombardelli G, Peruzzi G, Cattabeni F. In, Benzodiazepine Recognition Site Ligands: Biochemistry and Pharmacology (Biggio G and Costa E, eds.), 1985, pp. 227-237, Raven, New York.

2. Braestrup C, Nielsen M, Squires R. Life Sci 24:347-350, 1979.

3. Chiu TH, Rosenberg HC. Life Sci 23:1153-1158, 1978.

4. Corda MG, Giorgi O, Biggio G. Brain Res 384:60-67, 1986.

5. Corda MG, Giorgi O, Longoni B, Fernandez A, Biggio G. Adv Biochem Psychopharmacol 45:293-306, 1988.

6. Crawley JN, Marangos PJ, Stivers J, Goodwin FK. Neuropharmacology 21:85-89, 1982.

7. DiStefano P, Casse KR, Colello D, Boxman HB. Cell Biol Int Rep 3:163-167, 1979.

8. Farb DH, Borden LA, Chan CY, Czajkowski CM, Gibbs TT, Schiller GD. Ann NY Acad Sci 435:1-31, 1984.
9. File S. Psychopharmacology 77:284-288, 1982.
10. Frey HH, Phillipin HP, Scheuler W. Eur J Pharmacol 104:27-38, 1984.
11. Gallager DW, Lakoski JM, Gonsalfves SF, Rauch SL. Nature 308:74-77, 1984.
12. Gallager DW, Malcolm AB, Anderson SA, Gonsalves SF. Brain Res 342:26-36, 1985.
13. Gallager DW, Heninger C, Wilson MA. In, Allosteric Modulation of Amino Acid Receptors: Therapeutic Implications. Barnard EA and Costa E, eds. Raven Press Ltd., New York, 1989, p 91.
14. Greenblatt DJ, Shader RI. Drug Metab Rev 8:13-28, 1978.
15. Greenblatt DJ, Shader RI, Abernethy DR. N Engl J Med 309:410-416, 1983.
16. Haefely W, Kyburz E, Gerecke M, Möhler H. Adv Drug Res 14:165-322, 1985.
17. Haigh JRM, Feely M, Gent JP. J Pharm Pharmacol 38:931-934, 1986.
18. Heninger C, Gallager DW. Neuropharmacology 27:1073-1076, 1988.
19. Hess EJ, Albers LJ, Le H, Creese I. J Pharmacol Exp Ther 238:846-854, 1986.
20. Lister RG, File SE, Greenblatt DJ. Psychopharmacology 81:292-294, 1984.
21. Jong Y-J, Thampy KG, Barnes EM. Dev Brain Res 25:83-89, 1986.
22. Maloteaux J-M, Octave J-N, Gossuin A, Laterre C, Trouet A. Eur J Pharmacol 144:173-183, 1987.
23. Marley RJ, Gallager DW. Eur J Pharmacol 159:217-223, 1989.
24. Medina JH, Novas ML, Wolfman C, Destein ML, DeRobertis E. Neuroscience 9:331-335, 1983.
25. Medina JH, Novas ML, DeRobertis E. Eur J Pharmacol 90:125-128, 1983.
26. Miller LG, Greenblatt DJ, Barnhill JG, Shader RI. J Pharmacol Exp Ther 246:170-176, 1988.
27. Miller LG, Greenblatt DJ, Summer WR, Shader RI. J Pharmacol Exp Ther 246:177-182, 1988.
28. Miller LG, Greenblatt DJ, Roy RB, Gaver A, Lopez F, Shader RI. Upregulation of GABA$_A$ receptor binding and function associated with chronic benzodiazepine antagonist administration. J Pharmacol Exp Ther 248:1096-1101, 1989.
29. Miller LG, Woolverton S, Greenblatt DJ, Lopez F, Roy RB, Shader RI. Biochem Pharmacol (in press).
30. Miller LG, Roy RB, Weill CL. (submitted for publication)
31. Miller LG, Lopez F, Schatzki A, Heller J, Greenblatt DJ, Shader RI. (submitted for publication)
32. Möhler H, Okada T, Enna SJ. Brain Res 156:392-395, 1978.
33. Nutt DJ. Trends in Pharm Sci 7:457-460, 1986.

34. Overstreet DJ, Yamamura HI. Life Sci 25:1865-1877, 1979.
35. Reeves PM, Schweizer MP. Brain Res 270:376-379, 1983.
36. Roca DJ, Schiller GD, Farb DH. Molec Pharmacol 33:481-485, 1988.
37. Rosenberg HC, Chiu TH. Life Sci 24:803-808, 1979.
38. Rosenberg HG, Chiu TH. Eur J Pharmacol 70:435-460, 1981.
39. Rosenberg HC, Tietz EI, Chiu TH. Neuropharmacology 24:639-644, 1985.
40. Russell RW, Ehlert FJ, Hwa JJ. Psychopharmacology 88:33-39, 1986.
41. Scharf MB, Feil P. Life Sci 32:1771-1777, 1983.
42. Sher PK. Epilepsia 24:313-320, 1983.
43. Sher PK, Machen VL. Brain Dev 9:33-36, 1987.
44. Shibla DB, Gardell MA, Neale JH. Brain Res 210:471-474, 1981.
45. Spirt NM, Zanko M, Bautz G, O'Brien RA. Soc Neurosci Abstr 8:375, 1982.
46. Therani MHJ, Barnes EM. Dev Brain Res 25:91-100, 1986.
47. Thampy KG, Barnes EM. Biol Chem 259:1753-1757, 1984.
48. Tietz EI, Rosenberg HC, Chiu TH. J Pharmacol Exp Ther 236:384-391, 1986.
49. Treit D. Biochem Behav 22:383-387, 1985.
50. Woods JH, Katz JL, Winger G. Pharmacol Rev 39:251-413, 1987.
51. Yu O, Chiu TH, Rosenberg HC. J Pharmacol Exp Ther 246:107-113, 1988.

GABA and Benzodiazepine Receptor Subtypes,
edited by Giovanni Biggio and Erminio Costa.
Raven Press, New York © 1990.

HEPATIC ENCEPHALOPATHY:

NEUROCHEMICAL MECHANISMS AND NEW TREATMENTS

M. Baraldi, P. Zanoli and M.L. Zeneroli*

Cattedra di Farmacologia e Farmacognosia della Facolta' di
Farmacia, Dipartimento di Scienze Farmaceutiche e Cattedra di
Semeiotica Medica della Facolta' di Medicina*, Universita' di
Modena, 41100 Modena, Italy.

Hepatic encephalopathy (HE) which results from fulminant hepatic failure (FHF) or from chronic liver disease (PSE) is a neuropsychiatric syndrome characterized by abnormal mental status with changes in personality and intellectual capacity. This syndrome has been considered since always a metabolic disorder because it is potentially fully reversible (32); there are, however, many structural changes in both neurons and glial cells, described in the brain of both patients and animals, which might be considered as responsible of the progression of the neurological symptoms leading to consciousness disturbances and coma. Gliosis and neuronal necrosis with evidence of brain atrophy in HE due to FHF and to PSE have been described (1,12,16,25,36,48,49,50,58).

HE is considered secondary to accumulation, in extracellular fluids, of toxic products that have not been metabolized by the liver. Many pathogenetic agents, which seem to be mainly toxic metabolites of gut origin, have been proposed but all of them are still the subject of controversy. Among them, ammonia is often incriminated (60) as well as the plasma amino acid imbalance which leads to an increased presence in the brain of phenylalanine, thyrosine and free tryptophan (33). The increased presence of aromatic amino acids in the brain generated the "false neurotransmitter" hypothesis of HE (33). While the described increase of octopamine seems to be a secondary event in the develpoment of HE, the increased presence of tryptophan and of its metabolites, such as the quinolinic acid, has recently attracted interest. An increased presence in the brain of quinolinic acid, which is considered an excitatory neurotoxic amino acid, as been, in fact, described both in animal models and in patients with HE (37). In this context, however, an increased release of glutamic acid, the major excitatory amino acid in the brain, due to an hyperammoniemic state leading to an excessive presence of this amino acid in the extracellular space and in turn to degeneration processes

177

has been described in animal models of HE (37). Whatever the pathogenetic agents could be, since the early 1980's we suggested that HE could be regarded as a degenerative disorder. This concept was based on the evidence that in experimental models of HE due to FHF in rats (4,9) and of PSE in dogs (10,56,59) there was an increased functional activity of the GABA-A receptors which was interpreted as an expression of a denervation supersensitivity phenomenon. An increased GABAergic tone, using a rabbit model of HE due to FHF, has been described at the same time but with a different interpretation (44,45).

The GABA-A receptor is a large supramolecular entity which includes GABA recognition sites, Benzodiazepine recognition sites, chloride ionophore and endogenous modulators. In particular, the GABA-A receptor includes a beta subunit with binding sites for several compounds among which there are both the anxiolytic Benzodiazepines and the anxiogenic beta-carbolines. The finding that the GABA recognition sites were increased in the mild stage of HE due to FHF in rats coupled with the demonstration that the target enzyme of the GABA synthesis in nerve terminals, glutamic acid decarboxylase, was reduced (55) suggested us the presence, in this stage, of a denervation supersensitivity phenomenon due to degeneration processes. This concept, in fact, was in line with the described increase in the density of GABA receptors after chemical or surgically-induced lesions in brain areas of rats (30,51). The presence of degenerative phenomena seem to be corroborated by the finding that in rats with severe stage of HE, which is an agonal status, there is a loss of low affinity GABA receptors (4,9). The above mentioned alterations of GABA receptors in the two different stages of HE have been confirmed by studying the characteristics of GABA receptors solubilized from brain membranes of normal rats and of rats in mild and severe stage of HE (14).

It is known that Benzodiazepines act as positive allosteric modulators of GABAergic transmission, thereby increasing GABAergic activity and general central nervous system inhibition (21). Clinical observation in patients with acute or chronic liver diseases suggests that these patients are supersensitive to administration of sedatives and in particular of Benzodiazepines (2,18). This phenomenon, which has been attributed for some time, to an altered metabolism of Benzodiazepines in such patients, has been proved to be due also to an increased sensitivity of the central nervous system during HE. Studies performed both in rats with acute liver failure and in dogs with chronic liver disease using 3H-Diazepam and 3H-RO 15-1788 as radioligands showed an increased presence of Benzodiazepine recognition sites in brain membranes of animals in mild and in severe stage of HE (11,57). Since Benzodiazepine recognition sites are part of the GABA receptor complex, it is likely that the increase in Benzodiazepine receptors in comatose animals is attributable to a reactive compensatory phenomenon which might follow degenerative processes, as described for the GABA receptors. An increase in Benzo-

diazepine recognition sites has been described, in fact, after
kainic acid induced degeneration in brain (17). Indeed, in our
rat model we provided evidence of neuronal degeneration already
present in the mild stage of HE documented by rapid Golgi impre-
gnetion (12) and by electronmicroscopy (15).

The presence of degenerative processes in brain during experimental HE does not seem to be in conflict with the notion that
HE in man can be reversible probably because the central nervous
system can spontaneously recover from injury depending on the
substrates that support neurons survival and since degeneration
and regeneration of neurons may occur at the same time in pathological conditions (31). In this context it is noteworthy that
some of the rats can recover from the mild stage of HE thus
suggesting that the supersensitivity phenomenon of the GABAergic
system is reversible at this stage of HE.

A necessary requisite to show that these changes of receptors
during HE are operative in vivo is to perform pharmacological
challenges with both agonists and antagonists of GABA and Benzodiazepine in animals with HE.

PHARMACOLOGICAL CHALLENGE WITH GABA AGONISTS AND ANTAGONISTS IN RATS WITH MILD HE

HE was induced in Sprague-Dawley albino rats (125-150 g) by i.
p. injection of Galactosamine-HCl (3g/Kg) as previously described
(54). Briefly, the animals, which develop FHF as a result of
massive necrosis of the liver, within 48 hrs show a progressive
encephalopathy characterized in the mild stage by stupor an poor
righting reflex. The severe stage is characterized by a period of
unconsciousness, diminished response to pain and flaccidity which
leads to the death of the animals 3.5 - 4 days after the injection of the toxins. In the present study rats in the mild stage
of HE were selected in order to perform pharmacological studies.
A group of these animals were precannulated under light ether
anesthesia before the injection of the hepatoxin.

As shown in Table 1, the intracerebroventricular injection of
a dose of Muscimol (400 ng/rat), which induces only a motility
reduction in control rats, elicits, when injected in rats with
mild HE a complete loss of righting reflex. It is noteworthy
that, while control rats recover from the effect of Muscimol
within 3 hrs, 66 % of the rats with mild HE died within 3 hrs
after the Muscimol injection. These data seem to indicate that in
the early stage of HE there is an increased response to the
administration of GABA agonist, a finding which seems to corrobo-
rate the described increase of the GABAergic receptor system.

Since an increased tone of the GABAergic system seems to play
a key role in the generalized depression of the central nervous
system which characterizes HE, we thought that the use of GABA
antagonists could be of value in order to counteract the symptoms
of HE. The injection of the isosteric inhibitor of GABA receptors, Bicuculline, in rats with mild stage of HE rather than to

TABLE 1.   Effect of intracerebroventricular injection of Muscimol* in normal rats and in rats with mild stage of galactosamine induced HE.

Condition	Rats N.	Dose (ng/rat)		Behavior	Death rate % within 3 hr
Controls	10	saline		none	0
	10	muscimol	400	motility reduction	0
	10	muscimol	800	loss righting reflex	10
Mild HE	10	saline		drowisness	0
	10	muscimol	400	loss righting reflex	70
	10	muscimol	800	loss righting reflex	100

*Muscimol or saline were injected in a fixed volume of 5 ul to precannulated rats.

ameliorate the symptoms of HE precipitated the death of the animals (Table 2) by inducing tonic-clonic convulsions with an ED-100 which was 50 % lower of that of control rats. As a whole, the informations which derives from these pharmacological experiments seem to confirm the increased sensitivity of the GABAergic system in HE and to suggest that the increased functional activity of this system surmised from the biochemical experiments seems to be operative at least in this experimental model of HE. The demonstration that already at the onset of encephalopathy the rats showed an increased sensitivity to Bicuculline indicates that for a therapeutic point of view the use of isosteric antagonists of GABA receptors cannot be used because of the potential high risk for patients with HE to develop

TABLE 2.   Effect of intracerebroventricular injection of Bicucilline-methiodide in normal rats and in rats with mild stage of Galactosamine-induced HE.

Rats	Bicuculline* ED-100 (ng/rat)	Tonic-clonic convulsion %	Onset (sec)^	Duration of convulsive activity (min)	Death rate %
Controls	750	100	$19.2 + 4.2$	$18.0 + 5.6$	0
Mild HE	375	100	$15.0 + 8.0$	$11.2 + 7.8$	100

*Bicuculline was injected in a fixed volume of 5 ul to precannulated rats using increasing doses from 125 to 750 ng. Values are reported as ^mean $+$ SD

seizure episodes.

PHARMACOLOGICAL CHALLENGE WITH BENZODIAZEPINE AGONISTS AND ANTAGONISTS IN RATS WITH MILD HE

The demonstration that the number of Benzodiazepine recognition sites is increased in brain membranes of animals in the mild stage of HE in parallel with the increase in GABA recognition sites might indicate that the GABA-A receptor complex as a whole undergoes the same fate in this pathological condition. To prove that indeed our animals, were supersensitive to Benzodiazepine administration, as it appens in patients, we performed experiments by injecting in vivo Benzodiazepine receptor agonists such as Oxazepam or Diazepam, which is metabolized in the liver giving rise to active metabilites. In particular, as shown in Table 3, a dose of 5 mg/Kg of Diazepam, which in normal animals induced only a reduction in motor activity without producing loss of righting reflex or death, induced, when injected in rats with mild stage of HE, a complete loss of the righting reflex and death in 50 % of the animals within 3 hrs. In this context it is noteworthy that within the above considered time none of the rats in mild stage of HE, injected in parallel with saline, died because of the progression of HE, thus suggesting that indeed the administration of Diazepam precipitate the syndrome.

This notion seems to be confirmed by the data obtained with the injection of Oxazepam by performing dose-effect experiments in

TABLE 3. Effect of an agonist and of an antagonist of Benzo diazepine receptors administered to normal rats and to rats with mild stage of galactosamine induced HE.

Rats	Drug	Motility % of controls	Loss of righting reflex %	Death within 3 hr %
Controls	saline	100	0	0
	diazepam	52	0	0
	RO 15-1788	106	0	0
Mild HE	saline	53	0	0
	diazepam	0	100	50
	RO 15-1788	90	0	0

Diazepam (5 mg/Kg) was administered by oral route while RO 15-1788 (10 mg/kg) was intraperitoneally injected.
The motor activity was measured for 15 min within 30 and 60 min after the drug injection, using an electronic actimeter. Mean values ($\pm$ SD) of controls expressed as activity counts/rat/15 min were 3,727 $\pm$ 241.

TABLE 4. Increased sensitivity to Oxazepam administration in rats at the onset of the mild stage of galactosamine induced HE.

Conditions	ED-50 (mg/kg/os) (Motility reduction)
Control	3.8 ± 0.3
Mild HE	2.5 ± 0.1*

The motor activity was recorded as described in the legend of table 3. Values are reported as Mean $\pm$ SD. Student's t-Test: *$p < 0.01$ vs controls.

both normal animals and animals with a mild stage of HE in order to find out the ED-50 for the motor activity reduction. As shown in Table 4, the value of the ED-50 of Oxazepam in rats was practically 50 % reduced in rats at the onset of the mild stage in comparison with controls.

Considering these effects induced by the injection of positive allosteric modulators of the GABA-A receptors we thought that antibenzodiazepine compounds able to reduce the positive effect of Benzodiazepines on the GABA-A receptor functional activity could be of value in the attempt to counteract the supersensitivity of the GABAergic system in HE. The use of the benzodiazepine antagonist RO 15-1788 which, as shown in Table 3, when injected in normal animals did not show any appreciable effect on the spontaneous motor activity, was able to recover the motor activity impaired in rats with the mild stage of HE. This finding confirms and extends the results obtain by using another benzodiazepine antagonist, that is CGS 8216, which was described to counteract the symptoms of HE and to normalize the visual evoked potential recording of rats with HE (11).

CONCLUSIONS AND THERAPEUTIC PERSPECTIVES

From these studies it seems that an increased tone of the GABAergic system could play a key role in the generalized depression of the central nervous system wich mainly characterizes HE. This concept was supported by the biochemical, electrophysiological and pharmacological experiments performed in HE deriving from acute and chronic experimental liver disease. It must be mentioned, however, that changes in GABA-A receptors have been described in some but not all animal models of HE (34,35,44,53) and in one out of two studies performed in autopsied brain tissues from patients with HE (19,27).
Our original demonstration that benzodiazepine antagonists can temporarely antagonize the symptoms of HE seems to confirm the suggested pathology of the GABAergic system in HE and opened up a new way in the attempt to counteract the neurological disturbances of HE. Transfer of data from animal models to humans is

always critical. The use of RO 15-1788 (Flumazenil), however, administered to patients with HE, has been shown to increase their level of consciousness and to normalize their EEG pattern (3,28,46,47).

These positive effects of the antibenzodiazepine compounds in the treatment of HE awaits further confirmations by extensive clinical trials but there is no doubt that they have generated a new impact in the studies of the pathogenesis of HE.

Endogenous ligands with agonist properties on the Benzodiazepine receptors have been suggested to be implicated in HE (38). The increased GABAergic tone in HE could be the result of an increased stimulation of GABA-A receptors by endogenous Benzodiazepine-like compounds. Following this theory the improvement induced by the administration of benzodiazepine antagonists in the neurological symptoms of HE must be referred to their ability to inhibit the activity of increased levels of endogenous compounds active on the GABA-A receptors.

Several endogenous ligands for Benzodiazepine recognition sites have been suggested. Among them there are the polypeptide DBI (Diazepam binding inhibitor) (22) and the Benzodiazepine themselves (24). Recently trace amounts of Benzodiazepines have been found in human brain and in plasma (24) and evidence have been provided that the neuropeptide DBI, which is an endogenous negative allosteric modulator of GABA-A receptors, is present in brain tissue in high concentration (29). Changes in the level of this endogenous ligand could contribute to the altered functional activity of the GABAergic system in HE. So far, an increased presence of Benzodiazepine-like substances (39,40) and DBI-like peptides (42) has been described only in cerebrospinal fluid and in blood of encephalopathic patients. From these findings it has been speculated that endogenous ligands for Benzodiazepine receptors could play a pathogenetic role in HE by promoting GABAergic neurotransmission.

Bearing in mind that the pathogenetic agents and the neurochemical derangements must be considered, at least in this pathology, as different entities, further evidence must be provided before to consider the Benzodiazepine-like substances as the only pathogenetic factor of HE. On the other hand, pharmacological and electrophysiological demonstrations were provided that an increase of the GABAergic tone induced in normal animals even leading to an impaired motor function and to a decreased consciousness associated with changes in visula evoked potential recordings, does not completely mimic the changes observed in HE (54).

The generalized depression of the central nervous system wich characterizes HE, in fact, seems to be the result of an imbalance between an increased tone of the GABAergic system and a decreased functional activity of excitatory neurotransmission systems such as Dopamine (6) and Glutamate (20,26). While the decreased functional activity of the Dopaminergic system seems to be a contributory factor to the above mentioned imbalance, an altered functional activity of the Glutamatergic system could play an important role in the early stage of HE and could explain the neuronal degeneration since the neurotoxicity of this excitatory neurotransmitter has been well established (43). Changes in the density of Glutamate receptors has been described in acute and chronic models of HE (15,20,26) and experimental evidence have been provided that hyperammoniemia increases glutamate release (37) and up-regulate Glutamate receptors (26). An accumulation of glutamate in the extracellular space could be responsible of the degeneration processes described in HE.

The presence of degenerative phenomena in HE seems to be confirmed by the observation that there is a decreased content of zinc in brain tissue of rats during HE (5), an event wich seems attributable to profound changes in the intrinsic characteristics of biomembranes since this element is very tightly bound to intrinsic components of cell membranes. Moreover evidence have been provided that free zinc may modulate both the GABAergic and the Glutamatergic systems (7,8,13,41,52).

Following the idea that glutamate can play an important role in the neuronal degeneration which takes place during HE, the negative allosteric modulator of the NMDA-Glutamate receptors, GM-1 (23), was administered, in association with the administration of NGF, to rats with ongoing HE and this therapy proved to be able to minimize neuronal degeneration and to improve survival (15).

There are several problems to be solved to gain a complete understanding of the pathogenesis and of the neurochemical mechanisms of HE, but the results derived from all the above mentioned studies could favor the discovery of new possible treatments for HE.

REFERENCES

1. Adams, R.D., and Foley, J.M. (1953): Annu. Rev. Nerv. Ment. Dis. Proc., 32:198-215.
2. Bakti, G., Fish, H.U., Karlaganis, G. (1987): Hepatology, 7:629-638.
3. Bansky, G., Meier, P.I., Zeigler, W.H., Walzer, H., Schmid, M., Huber, M. (1985): Lancet, 1:1324-1325.
4. Baraldi, M., Zeneroli, M.L. (1982): Science, 216:427-429.
5. Baraldi, M., Caselgrandi, E., Borella, P., Zeneroli, M.L. (1983). In: Application of behavioral pharmacology in toxicology, edited by C. Zbinden, V. Cuomo, C. Racagni, pp. 243-250, Raven Press, New York.
6. Baraldi, M., Zeneroli, M.L., Ricci, P., Ventura, E. (1983): Life Sci., 32:1417-1425.
7. Baraldi, M., Caselgrandi, E., Santi, M. (1984): In: The neurobiology of zinc (part A), edited by C.J. Frederickson, G.A. Howel, E.J. Kasarkis, E.J. (eds), pp 59-71. Alan R. Liss, New York.
8. Baraldi, M., Pinelli, G., Ricci, P., Zeneroli, M.L. (1984):

In: The neurobiology of zinc (part B), edited by C.J. Frederickson, G.A. Howel, E.J. Kasarkis, pp. 291-306. Alan R. Liss, New York.

9. Baraldi, M., Zeneroli, M.L. (1984): In: Dynamics of neuro transmitter function, edited by H. Hanin, pp. 349-356, Raven Press, New York.

10. Baraldi, M., Zeneroli, M.L., Ventura, E., Pinelli,G., Ricci, P., Santi, M., Racagni, G., Iuliano, E., Casciarri, I., Germini, M., Cavalletti, E., Tofanetti, O. (1984): In: Advances in hepatic encephalopathy and urea cycle diseases, edited by G. Kleinberger, P. Ferenci, P. Rieder, H. Thaler, pp. 353-359, Karger, Basel.

11. Baraldi, M., Zeneroli, M.L., Ventura, E., Penne, A., Pinelli, G., Ricci, P., Santi, M. (1984): Clin. Sci., 67:167-175.

12. Baraldi, M., Della Giustina, E., Botticelli, A.R. (1986): Falk Symposium, N. 44, 240.

13. Baraldi, M., Zanoli, P., Benelli, A., Sandrini, M., Giberti, A., Caselgrandi, E., Tosi, G., Preti, C. (1986): In: Excitatory aminoacids and epilepsy, edited by R. Schwarcz and Y. Ben-Ari, Y., pp. 571-585, Plenum Press, New York.

14. Baraldi, M., Massotti, M., Zeneroli, M.L. (1988): In: Advances in ammonia metabolism and hepatic encephalopathy. edited by P.B. Soeters, J.H.P. Wilson, A.J. Meijer, E. Holm, pp.238-242, Excerpta Medica, Amsterdam.

15. Baraldi, M., Zanoli, P., Zeneroli, M.L., Fano, R.A., Fante, R., Trentini, G.P. (1989): Soc. Neurosci., 369.18.

16. Bernthal, P., Hays, A., Tarter, R.E., Van Thield, D., Lecky, J., Hegedus, A. (1987): Hepatology, 7:107-114.

17. Biggio, G., Corda, M.G., Concas, A., Gessa, G.L. (1981): Brain Res., 220:344-349.

18. Branch, R.A., Morgan, M.H., James, J., and Read, A.E. (1976), Gut, 17:975-983.

19. Butterworth, R.F., Lavoie, J., Giguere, J.F., and Pomier-Layrargues, G. (1988.): Hepatology, 8:1084-1088.

20. Butterworth, R.F., Lavoie, J., Szerb, J.C., Peterson, C., Cotman, C.W. (1988): Proceedings of International symposium on Hepatic encephalopathy: pathophysiology and treatment, Canada, Abs. 10.

21. Costa, E. and Guidotti, A. (1979): Ann.Rev. Pharmacol. Toxi col., 19:531-545.

22. Costa, E., and Guidotti, A. (1987): In: Psychopharmacology: the third generation of progress. edited by H.Y. Meltzer, pp. 425-435, Raven Press, New York.

23. Costa, E., Alho, H., Favaron, M., Manev, H. (1989): In: Allosteric modulation of amino acid receptors: therapetic implications. edited by E.A. Barnard, E. Costa, pp. 3-18, Raven Press, New York.

24. DeBlas, A.L. (1988): TINS, 11:489-490.

25. Diemer, N.H. (1978): Acta Neurol.Scand., 58 (suppl 71):1-143.

26. Ferenci, P., Pappas, S.C., Munson, P.J., Jones, A.E. (1984): Hepatology, 4:25-29.

27. Ferenci, P., Riederer, P., Jellinger, K., Schafer, D.F., Jones, E.A. (1988): Liver, 8:225-230.
28. Ferenci, P., Grimm, G., Meryn ,S., Gangl, A. (1989): Gastroenterology, 96:240-243.
29. Ferrero, P., Costa, E., Conti-Tronconi, B., and Guidotti, A. (1986): Brain Res., 399:136-142.
30. Gale, K., and Iadarola, M.J. (1980): Brain Res., 183:217-223.
31. Graveland, G.A., Williams, R.S., Difiglia, M. 1985. Science, 227:770-773.
32. Hoyumpa, A.M., and Schenker, S. (1982): J. Lab. Clin. In vest., 100:477-487.
33. James, J.H., Ziparo, V., Jeppson, B., Fischer, J.E. (1979): Lancet, 2: 772-775.
34. Maddison, J.E., Dodd, P.R.,Johnston, J.A.R., Farrell, G.C. (1987): Gastroenterlogy, 93:1062-1068.
35. Maddison, J.E., Dodd, P.R., Morrison, M., Johnston, G.A.R., Farrel, G.C. (1987): Hepatology, 7:621-628.
36. Martinez, A. (1968): Acta Neuropathol., 11:82-86.
37. Moroni, F., Carla', V., Lombardi, G., Pellegrini, D., Carassale, G.L., Cortesini, C. (1984): In: Advances in hepatic encephalopathy and urea cycle diseases, edited by G. Kleinberger, P. Ferenci, P. Rieder, H. Thaler, pp. 385-393, Karger, Basel.
38. Mullen, K.D., Martin, J.V., Mendelson, W.B., Bassett, M.L., Jones, E.A. (1988): Lancet 1:457-459.
39. Mullen, K.D., Szauter, K.M., Kaminsky, K., Tolentino, P.D. (1988): Hepatology, 8:1254.
40. Olasmaa, M., Guidotti, A., Costa, E., Rothstein,J.D., Goldman, M.E., Weber, R.J., Paul, S.M. (1989): Lancet, 1:491-492.
41. Peters, S., Koh, J., Choi, D.W. (1987): Science, 236:589-592.
42. Rothstein, J.D., Mckhann, G., Guarnieri, P., Barbaccia, A., Guidotti, A., Costa, E.(1989): Ann. Neurol., (in press).
43. Rothman, S.M. and Olney, J.W. (1987): TINS, 10:299-302.
44. Schafer, D.F., and Jones, A.E. (1982): Lancet, 1:18-20.
45. Schafer, D.F., Fowler, J.M., Munson, P.J., Thakur, A.K., Waggoner J.G., Jones, E.A. (1983): J. Lab. Clin. Med., 102:870-880.
46. Scollo-Lavizzari, G. (1985): Lancet, 1:1324.
47. Sutherland, L.R., Minuk, G.Y. (1988): Ann. Int. Med., 108:158.
48. Toda, C., Chiba, T., Matsuda, Y., Imatome, T., Inoh, T., Fujita, T.(1983): Am. J. Gastroenterol., 78:446-447.
49. Tubbs, H., Parker, J.D., Murray-Lyon, L.M., and Williams, R. (1977): Med. Chir. Dig., 6:75-77.
50. Victor, M., Adams, R, Cole M. (1965): Medicine, 44:345-396.
51. Waddington, J.I., and Cross, A.J. (1978): Nature, 276:618 -620.
52. Westbrook, G.L., Mayer, M.L. (1987): Nature, 328:640-643.
53. Wysmyk-Cybula, U., Dabrowiexki, Z., Albrecht, J. (1986): Biomed. Biochim. Acta, 3:413-419.

54. Zeneroli, M.L., Penne, A., Parrinello, G., Cremonini, C., Ventura, E. (1981): Life Sci., 28:1507-1515.
55. Zeneroli, M.L., Iuliano, E., Racagni, C., Baraldi, M. (1982): J. Neurochem., 33:1219-1222.
56. Zeneroli, M.L., Baraldi, M., Pinelli, G., Grandi, S., Vezzelli, C., Contrucci, L., Penne, A., Ventura, E. (1984): In: Advances in hepatic encephalopathy and urea cycle diseases, edited by G. Kleinberger, P. Ferenci, P. Rieder, H. Thaler, pp. 94-106, Karger, Basel.
57. Zeneroli, M.L., Baraldi, M., Pinelli, G., Casciarri, I., Germini, M., Cavalletti, E., Tofanetti, O., Ventura, E. (1985): Hepatology, 5:953.
58. Zeneroli, M.L., Cioni, G., Vezzelli, C., Grandi, S., Crisi, G., Luzietti, R., Ventura, E. (1987): J. Hepatol., 4:283-292.
59. Zeneroli, M.L. and Baraldi, M. (1988): Hepatology, 8:1388.
60. Zieve, L. (1981): Hepatology, 1:360-365.

GABA and Benzodiazepine Receptor Subtypes,
edited by Giovanni Biggio and Erminio Costa.
Raven Press, New York © 1990.

THE INVOLVEMENT OF THE BENZODIAZEPINE RECEPTOR IN HEPATIC ENCEPHALOPATHY: EVIDENCE FOR THE PRESENCE OF A BENZODIAZEPINE RECEPTOR LIGAND.

Anthony S. Basile[1], Nancy L. Ostrowski[2], Sergio H. Gammal[3], E. Anthony Jones[3], and Phil Skolnick[1]

[1]Section on Neurobiology, Laboratory of Neuroscience, NIDDK, [2]Section on Clinical Brain Imaging, Laboratory of Cerebral Metabolism, NIMH, and [3]Liver Diseases Section, Digestive Diseases Branch, NIDDK, National Institutes of Health, Bethesda, MD

Hepatic encephalopathy (HE) is a neuropsychiatric disorder that complicates acute (due to viral hepatitis or drug overdose) or chronic (due to alcoholic cirrhosis or chronic hepatitis) liver failure[10,13,23,26]. HE is characterized in humans by a sequential degradation of mentation and neuromuscular function. The neuropsychiatric and neuromuscular manifestations can be classified into four clinical stages: I - confusion, mild incoordination; II-drowsiness, asterixis, ataxia; III - stupor, inarticulate speech, hyperreflexia, muscle rigidity; IV - coma, loss of oculovestibular responses[3,26]. HE is not associated with alterations in CNS architecture, and is a potentially reversible metabolic encephalopathy regardless of the nature of the underlying liver dysfunction. This syndrome is a major public health problem worldwide, and it would be highly desirable to develop a therapeutic regimen to ameliorate the symptoms at the target organ of this syndrome-the brain.

Despite extensive investigation, the pathogenesis of this syndrome is unclear. Recently, evidence has accumulated indicating that increased GABAergic neurotransmission may account for some of the behavioral and electrophysiological manifestations of HE in several animal models and humans[7,14-16,21,22]. This hypothesis is based on the observation that enhancement of inhibitory neurotransmitter tone in the CNS can cause the ataxia, sedation and coma observed in HE, and may explain in part the increased sensitivity of patients with chronic liver failure to benzodiazepines[1,9].

THE GALACTOSAMINE-TREATED RABBIT MODEL OF FULMINANT HEPATIC FAILURE

The hypothesis that the GABAergic neurotransmitter system is involved in HE is based, in part, on observations of changes in the gross electrical activity of an animal model of HE, the galactosamine-treated rabbit model of fulminant hepatic failure (FHF). This model closely resembles HE due to FHF in humans with respect to the development of neuromuscular deficits observed in HE[8,13]. Within 24-48 hr. after the administration of a single dose (4.3 mmol/kg IV) of galactosamine (a selective hepatotoxin showing no CNS toxicity), the rabbit develops a series of readily staged decrements in neuromuscular function (Table 1). These neuromuscular function abnormalities strongly indicate

Table 1. Behavioral characteristics of the galactosamine-treated rabbit model of hepatic encephalopathy

----

Stage 1: Sedation, lack of responsiveness to stimuli

Stage 2: Mild ataxia, poor head posture

Stage 3: Severe ataxia, hindlimb extension, loss of righting reflex, loss of flexor tonus, nystagmus

Stage 4: Coma

----

the presence of a cerebellar deficit. Within 6 hours after the initiation of these symptoms the rabbit becomes comatose and dies. Other than mild edema, there are no gross pathological changes in the brains of these animals. Concurrent with the motor function abnormalities in these rabbits are significant changes in the pattern of the visual evoked responses[7,22]. These changes could be mimicked by agents that increase GABAergic tone, and are normalized by $GABA_A$ and benzodiazepine (BZ) receptor antagonists. Since the VER represents an average of the electrical activity of large and poorly defined neuronal populations in the occipital cortex and subcortical regions, ascribing the changes in CNS activity observed in HE to alterations in the function of a specific neurotransmitter system with confidence requires a technique capable of monitoring neuronal activity with higher resolution. One complementary technique is to record changes in the electrical activity of single neurons in response to exposure to pharmacologic agents specific for the supramolecular

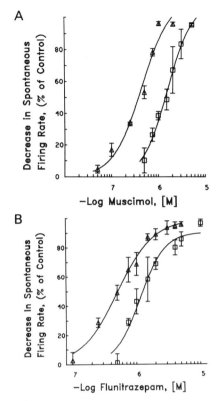

FIG 1. Concentration-response curves for the inhibition of Purkinje neuron activity by muscimol (A) and flunitrazepam (B). Symbols:(open triangles), HE neurons; (open squares), control neurons. The IC_{50} values of muscimol for control and HE neurons are 1.37 and 0.30 μM, respectively. The IC_{50} values for flunitrazepam for control and HE curves are 1.71 and 0.50 μM, respectively.

complex. In view of the pronounced cerebellar deficits seen in the rabbit model of HE, the spontaneous activity of Purkinje neurons was recorded from cerebellar slices maintained in vitro[2].

NEURONS FROM RABBITS WITH HE ARE ACTIVATED BY BENZODIAZEPINE RECEPTOR ANTAGONISTS.

Using rabbit cerebellar slices maintained in vitro, the spontaneous activity of Purkinje neurons from rabbits with HE due to FHF was found to be 3-5 times more sensitive to depression by muscimol and flunitrazepam than that of control rabbit Purkinje neurons[5] (Figure 1). In contrast, Purkinje neurons from rabbits with HE were excited by the administration of the BZ receptor antagonists flumazenil and

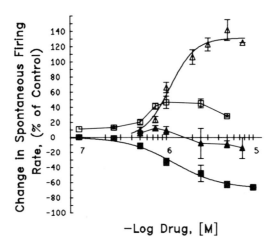

−Log Drug, [M]

FIG 2.   Concentration-response curves demonstrating the effects
of BZ receptor antagonists on Purkinje neuron activity.
Symbols: closed square, Control + Ro 15-1788; closed triangle,
Control + Ro 14-7437; open square, HE + Ro 15-1788; open
triangle, HE + Ro 14-7437.   Ro 15-1788 slightly decreased
control Purkinje neuron spontaneous activity (IC_{50} = 1.5 μM).
However, in Purkinje neurons from rabbits with HE, Ro 15-1788
increased the firing rate (EC_{50} = 0.35 μM).   Note that at the
highest concentration of Ro 15-1788 tested (5 μM), the
excitatory response of Purkinje neurons from rabbits with HE
declines.   In contrast, Ro 14-7437 had no effect on control
rabbit Purkinje neuron activity (0.5 - 7.5 μM) but elicited a
robust increase in spontaneous activity of Purkinje neurons
from rabbits with HE (IC_{50} = 1.43 μM).

Ro 14-7437 at concentrations which had no effect on, or
depressed the activity of control rabbit Purkinje neurons
(Figure 2).   Pretreating HE rabbit Purkinje neurons with a
subthreshold concentration of the BZ receptor antagonist Ro 14-
7437 eliminated the hypersensitivity of neurons from rabbits
with HE to depression by muscimol (Figure 3).   Finally, the
hypersensitivity of Purkinje neurons to depression appeared
specific for those agents acting at the supramolecular complex,
as no difference in the sensitivity of these neurons was seen
in response to treatment with phenylephrine, a depressant

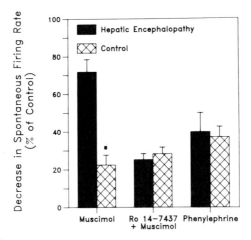

Drug Treatment

FIG 3.   The BZ antagonist Ro 14-7437 reverses the
hypersensitivity to muscimol-induced depression of Purkinje
neurons from rabbits with HE.   Purkinje neurons from rabbits
with HE were significantly more sensitive to depression by
muscimol (0.75μM) alone than control rabbit Purkinje neurons
(left bars).   However, pretreatment of Purkinje neurons from
rabbits with HE with a subthreshold concentration of Ro 14-7437
(0.5μM) reduced the subsequent muscimol-induced depression to
levels indistinguishable from those occurring in control rabbit
neurons (center bars).   In addition, this bargraph illustrates
the specificity of the differential sensitivity of Purkinje
neurons from rabbits with HE to depression by agents acting at
the GABA-benzodiazepine receptor (right bars).   Application of
phenylephrine (50μM) depressed the spontaneous activity of
Purkinje neurons from controls and rabbits with HE to a similar
extent.   * = Significantly different from all other groups, 2-
way ANOVA, p < 0.001.

alpha-adrenergic receptor agonist (Figure 3).
     The above electrophysiological observations clearly
implicate the GABA-BZ receptor complex in the pathogenesis of
HE.   Further, they suggest that BZ receptor antagonists may be
useful in reversing the encephalopathy.   However, it is not
clear what mechanism is responsible for these observations in

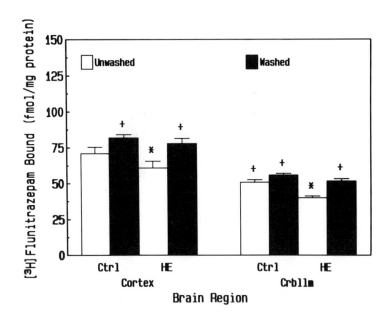

FIG 4. [³H]Flunitrazepam (1 nM) binding to laminae I-IV of the cerebral cortex (left bars) and cerebellar cortex (right bars) of control and HE rabbits. Adjacent sections were either washed for 30 minutes prior to incubation with radioligand (solid bars), or incubated with radioligand without prewashing (open bars). Unwashed sections from rabbits with HE showed significantly lower densities of [³H]flunitrazepam binding in laminae I-IV of the cerebral cortex (22%, 26% vs washed HE and control groups, respectively) and in the cerebellar cortex (24%, 30%, 22% vs washed HE and control and unwashed control groups, respectively). * = significantly different, p <0.05, Student-Newman-Keuls' Multiple Range Test after ANOVA, compared to groups labelled +.

Purkinje neurons from rabbits with HE. Although an increase inthe density and/or affinity of either the GABA or BZ receptors could account for the hypersensitivity of the Purkinje neurons from rabbits with HE to depression by muscimol or flunitrazepam, this would not explain the excitatory responses to administration of the BZ receptor antagonists. Alternatively, an increase in the concentration or availability of either GABA or a ligand for the BZ receptor with agonist properties could explain the hypersensitivity to depression of the HE rabbit neurons. Increases in plasma GABA concentrations have been reported in HE, although this issue remains controversial[11,12,17,18,20]. However, even if GABA levels were elevated in the CNS of rabbits with HE, this would explain the neuronal hypersensitivity to depressants, but not the excitations produced by BZ receptor antagonists. However, the presence of a BZ receptor agonist in HE could explain not only the excitatory responses to flumazenil, but also the hypersensitivity of these neurons to depressants acting at the supramolecular complex. Subsequent autoradiographic studies were performed to test these hypotheses.

AUTORADIOGRAPHIC STUDIES OF THE GABA-BZ RECEPTOR COMPLEX IN HEPATIC ENCEPHALOPATHY

Autoradiographic analysis was used to examine radioligand binding to BZ and $GABA_A$ receptors in the brains of rabbits with HE[6]. Thin sections of whole brain from HE and normal rabbits were mounted on slides and subdivided into two groups. One group was washed before incubation with radioligand, while the second group was not prewashed. [^{3}H]Flunitrazepam binding (Figure 4) to unwashed HE rabbit sections was significantly reduced ($p < 0.05$) by 22-26% in layers I-IV of the cerebral cortex, and by 22-30% in the cerebellar cortex. A similar, significant ($p < 0.05$) decrease in [^{3}H]Ro 15-1788 binding density to BZ receptors was also observed in the cerebral cortex (27-37%) and cerebellar cortex (26-33%) of unwashed HE rabbit sections (Figure 5).

Co-incubation of sections with [^{3}H]flunitrazepam in the presence of 100 μM muscimol and 200 mM NaCl increased radioligand binding to the cerebral and cerebellar cortices of control group sections by approximately 30 to 50% ($p < 0.05$, Figure 6). In contrast [^{3}H]flunitrazepam binding to the cerebral and cerebellar cortices was either unchanged or further decreased in sections from HE rabbits.

No differences in the binding of either [^{3}H]muscimol (Figure 6) or [^{3}H]PK 11195 were observed in the cerebral or cerebellar cortices among any of the control or HE rabbit groups analyzed.

These observations indicate the presence in situ of a reversible inhibitor of radioligand binding to the BZ receptor with agonist properties in the brains of rabbits with HE. This substance appears to be specific for the BZ receptor. Further, there is no evidence of change in the density of BZ or GABA receptors in HE.

NEUROCHEMICAL STUDIES INDICATE THE PRESENCE OF A BENZODIAZEPINE RECEPTOR LIGAND IN HEPATIC ENCEPHALOPATHY

Radioligand binding studies of the GABA and BZ receptor complex were performed in well-washed membranes from the cortex and cerebellum of normal and HE rabbits using the radioligands [^{3}H]SR 95531 for the GABA receptor, [^{3}H]Ro 15-1788 for the

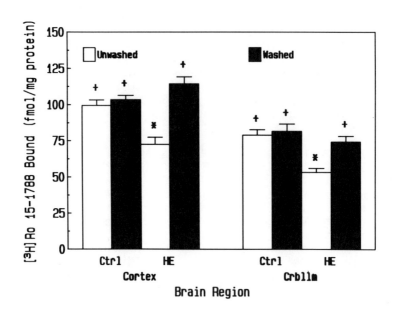

FIG 5. [³H]Ro 15-1788 (1 nM) binding to layers I-IV of the
cerebral cortex (left bars) and cerebellar cortex (right bars)
of control and HE rabbits.   Symbols are identical to those in
Figure 4.   Unwashed sections from rabbits with HE showed
significantly lower densities of [³H]Ro 15-1788 binding in
laminae I-IV of the cerebral cortex (37%, 30%, and 27%
vs washed HE and control, and unwashed control groups,
respectively) and in the cerebellar cortex (28%, 35%, 32% vs
washed HE and control and unwashed control groups,
respectively). * = significantly different, $p < 0.05$, Student-
Newman-Keuls' Multiple Range Test after ANOVA, compared to
groups labelled +.

BZ receptor, and [³⁵S]TBPS for the chloride ionophore.   Neither
the K_d nor the B_{max} for the binding of the above radioligands
to their respective receptors was changed in the cerebellum or
cerebral cortex of rabbits with HE.   Further, no changes in
the ability of NaCl, GABA or NaCl (200 mM) and GABA
(100 µM) together to enhance [³H]flunitrazepam binding to BZ
receptors in well-washed preparations of cerebellum and
cerebral cortex from normal rabbits and rabbits with HE was
observed.   These observations are consistent with the results

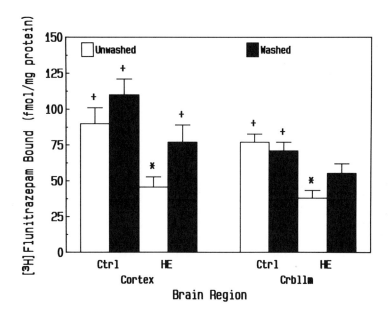

FIG 6. The effects of muscimol (100 μM) and NaCl (200 mM) on [³H]flunitrazepam (1 nM) binding to layers I-IV of the cerebral cortex (left bars) and cerebellar cortex (right bars) of control and HE rabbits. Symbols are identical to those in Figure 4. Unwashed sections from rabbits with HE showed significantly lower densities of [³H]flunitrazepam binding in laminae I-IV of the cerebral cortex (41%, 59%, 49% vs washed HE and control, and unwashed control groups, respectively) and in the cerebellar cortex (47%, 51% vs washed and unwashed control groups, respectively). * = significantly different, p <0.05, Student-Newman-Keuls' Multiple Range Test after ANOVA, compared to groups labelled +.

of previous electrophysiologic and autoradiographic studies indicating that no significant changes in the components of the GABA-BZ receptor supramolecular complex occur in HE.

Extracts of HE rabbit brain yielded high levels of a substance which inhibited the binding of [³H]Ro 15-1788 to BZ receptors in well-washed membranes from normal rabbit cerebral cortex. This inhibition was competitive and reversible. Further, the inhibition of [³H]Ro 15-1788 and [³H]flunitrazepam binding by extracts of HE rabbit brain could be enhanced by the addition of GABA and NaCl. Subsequent purification of

HE rabbit brain extracts using reverse-phase HPLC techniques yielded several fractions with inhibitory activity. Three of these fractions correlated with peaks of UV absorption having the same retention times as the BZ receptor agonists desmethyldiazepam, diazepam and oxazepam.

SUMMARY AND CONCLUSIONS

The involvement of GABAergic systems in the pathogenesis of HE was supported by electrophysiologic studies of single Purkinje neurons from rabbits with HE which demonstrated the hypersensitivity of these neurons to depression by GABA and BZ receptor agonists. In contrast, these neurons were excited by BZ receptor antagonists. At concentrations which had no effect on neuronal activity, BZ receptor antagonists also reversed the hypersensitivity of HE neurons to depression by muscimol. This combination of neuronal responses is consistent with an increase in the concentration or availability of a ligand for the BZ receptor with agonist properties in the brains of rabbits with HE.

Subsequent neurochemical studies support these electrophysiologic observations. Autoradiographic techniques indicated the presence of a reversible inhibitor of [^{3}H]Ro 15-1788 and [^{3}H]flunitrazepam binding to the cerebral and cerebellar cortices of rabbits with HE. The ability of this substance to inhibit [^{3}H]flunitrazepam binding to HE rabbit brain sections was further enhanced in the presence of NaCl and GABA. The autoradiographic studies suggested that the density and affinity of the components of the GABA-BZ receptor complex are unaltered in this animal model of HE. This inference is fully supported by the subsequent studies of radioligand binding to well-washed membrane preparations. Finally, extracts of HE rabbit brains yielded a family of substances with the properties of BZ receptor agonists. These substances may include, but are not limited to, diazepam, oxazepam and desmethyldiazepam, but do not include substances commonly elevated in the plasma and CSF of patients with HE[4].

The positive identification of these substances awaits confirmation by mass-spectroscopic analysis. However, the precedent for the presence of a family of benzodiazepines in animals that were not administered these drugs has been set. The origin of these substances is a matter of ongoing research. Several studies have shown the presence of benzodiazepines in plant and animal materials[24,25]. It is possible that these "endogenous" benzodiazepines are the result of contamination of the food chain. A normally functioning liver would capture and metabolize these compounds after their absorption from the gut. This function of the liver would be impaired in liver failure, thus allowing sufficient levels of BZ receptor agonists to accumulate in the CNS, contributing to the pathogenesis of HE. However, studies by DeBlas and coworkers have reported that 1,4 benzodiazepines are present in human brains preserved prior to the commercial use of these compounds[19]. Further, they have found benzodiazepines in cell lines cultured without potential exogenous sources of benzodiazepines. Thus, there are alternatives to the environmental contamination hypothesis for the origin of these compounds.

Given that benzodiazepines (and cyclopyrrolones) have been found in crop plants such as wheat and potatoes[24,25], it is not surprising that they might be incorporated into foodstuffs and absorbed into the body. Alternatively, benzodiazepines or their precursors may be synthesized by gut bacteria. Following their absorption, the precursors might be converted into active compounds. Finally, it is possible that BZ receptor agonists are synthesized endogenously. Although the last possibility may be the least likely contributor to the BZ receptor agonists that are elevated in HE, each of these hypotheses must be rigorously tested.

Regardless of the origin of the BZ receptor agonists associated with HE, their precise role in the pathogenesis of · this disorder remains to be determined. Although the presence of elevated levels of BZ receptor ligands appears to be clearly associated with HE, studies of the time course of the development of the syndrome and the appearance of these BZ receptor ligands remain to be undertaken. Nonetheless, the present studies provide a rational basis for the therapeutic intervention of the syndrome using BZ receptor antagonists. These investigations, in concert with neurochemical, electrophysiological and behavioral studies in both a rat model of HE and uncontrolled human trials, indicate that BZ receptor antagonists (such as flumazenil) may be of value in the rapid and effective management of HE.

Bibliography

1. Bakti, G., Fisch, H.U., Karlaganis, G., Minder, C., and Bircher, J. (1987): Hepatology, 9:629-638.
2. Basile, A.S., and Dunwiddie, T.V. (1984): Brain Res., 296:15-25.
3. Basile, A.S., and Gammal, S.H. (1988): Clin. Neuropharm.,11:401-422.
4. Basile, A.S., Gammal, S.H., Jones, E.A., and Skolnick, P. (1989): J. Neurochem., (in press).
5. Basile, A.S., Gammal, S.H., Mullen, K.D., Jones, E.A., and Skolnick, P. (1988): J. Neurosci., 8:2414-2421.
6. Basile, A. S., Ostrowski, N. L., Gammal, S.H., Jones, E.A., and Skolnick, P. (1989): Neuropsychopharmacol., (in press).
7. Bassett, M.L., Mullen, K.., Skolnick, P., and Jones, E.A. (1987): Gastroenterology, 93:1069-1077.
8. Blitzer, B.L., Waggoner, J.G., Jones, E.A., Gralnick, H., Towne, D., Butler, J., Weise, V., Kopin, I., Walters, I., Teychenne, P.F., Goodman, D.G., and Berk, P. (1978): Gastroenterology, 74: 664-671.

9. Branch, R.A., Morgan, M.H., Jones, J., and Read, A.E. (1976): Gut, 17: 975-983.
10. Conn, H.O., and Liebethal, M.M. (1978): The Hepatic Coma Syndromes and Lactulose. Williams & Wilkins, Baltimore.
11. Ferenci, P., Covell, D., Schafer, D.F., Waggoner, J.G., Shrager, R., and Jones, E.A. (1983): Hepatology, 3:507-512.
12. Hoyumpa, A.M. (1986): Hepatology, 6: 1042-1044.
13. Jones E.A., and Gammal, S.H. (1988): In: The Liver: Biology and Pathobiology, edited by I.A. Arias, W.B. Jakoby, H. Popper, D. Schacter, and D.A. Shafritz. pp. 985-1006. Raven Press, New York.
14. Jones, D.B., Mullen, K.D., Roessle, M., Maynard, T. and Jones, E.A. (1987): J. Hepatol., 4: 118-126.
15. Jones, E.A. and Schafer, D.F. (1986): In: Progress in Liver Diseases, edited by H. Popper and F. Schaffner. vol 8, pp 525-540, Grune & Stratton, New York.
16. Jones, E.A., Schafer, D.F., Ferenci, P. and Pappas, S.C. (1984): Hepatology, 4:1235-1242.
17. Levy, L.J., Leek, J. and Losowsky, M.S. (1987): Clin. Sci., 73:531-534.
18. Minuk, G.Y., Winder, A., Burgess, E.D., and Sargeant, E.J. (1985): Hepatogastroenterology, 32:171-174.
19. Sangameswaran, L., Fales, H.M., Friedrich, P., and DeBlas, A. (1986): Proc. Natl. Acad. Sci. 83: 9236-9240.
20. Schafer, D.F., Fowler, J.M., Brody, E., and Jones, E.A. (1980): Gastroenterology, 79:1052.
21. Schafer, D.F., and Jones, E.A. (1982): In: Progress in Liver Diseases, edited by H. Popper and F. Schaffner, Vol 7, pp 615-627, Grune & Stratton, New York.
22. Schafer, D.F., Pappas, S.C., Brody, L.E., Jacobs, R. and Jones, E.A. (1984): Gastroenterology, 86: 540-545.
23. Sherlock, S. (1985): In: Diseases of the Liver and Biliary System, edited by S. Sherlock, Seventh Edition, pp 91-107, Blackwell Scientific, Boston.
24. Wildmann, J., H. Mohler, W. Vetler, V. Ranalder, K. Schmidt, and R. Maurer (1987): J.Neural Transm. 70: 383-388.
25. Wildmann, J., Vetter, W., Ranalder, U.B., Schmidt, K., Maurer, R., and Mohler, H. (1988): Bioch. Pharmacol. 37:3549-3559.
26. Zieve, L. (1987): In: Diseases of the Liver, edited by L. Schiff and E.R. Schiff, Fifth Edition, pp 925-947, J.B. Lippincott, Philadelphia.

GABA and Benzodiazepine Receptor Subtypes,
edited by Giovanni Biggio and Erminio Costa.
Raven Press, New York © 1990.

ON THE PROCESSING OF DIAZEPAM BINDING INHIBITOR (DBI)
IN HUMAN BRAIN

P. GUARNERI, A. GUIDOTTI, and E. COSTA

FIDIA-Georgetown Institute   for the Neurosciences
Georgetown University, School of Medicine,
3900 Reservoir Road, N.W.,
Washington D.C. 20007, U.S.A.

During the last ten years, neuropeptide research has contributed
substantially to the growth of neuroscience by elucidating that
many neuropeptides coexist with classical neurotransmitters in
the same neuron and act as modulator of the primary transmitter
action in central and peripheral nervous systems (24). These
findings have changed the old concept that at a given synapse
neuronal communication is transacted by a single chemical signal
(11). In line with these new vistas, the information now
available strongly supports the idea that many synapses function
by utilizing multiple chemical signals and that in the event of
polytypic signaling involving neuropeptides these neuroactive
compounds function either as primary transmitters or as
modulators of the primary transmitter action. In this context,
the term primary transmitter is assigned to the signal that is
transduced into a message for the postsynatic cell, while the
term modulator indicates signals that act by changing the
probability of the primary transmitter action.
It is generally accepted that the neuropeptides involved in the
synaptic transaction of information are processing products of
larger precursor molecules (12). These precursors undergo
specific proteolytic cleavages and posttranslational
modifications which are critical steps for determining their
biological activity.

201

DBI AS A MODULATOR OF GABAergic SYNAPSES

DBI is a neuropeptide discovered by monitoring the ability of brain extracts to displace diazepam from specific high affinity recognition sites located in brain membranes (1,6,19,33). This neuropeptide has a molecular weight of about 11 kDa and in rat brain coexists with GABA in the same GABAergic neurons (23,15). In primary cultures of mouse spinal cord neurons, DBI negatively modulates GABAergic transmission (8,9). "In vivo" it functions as the precursor for a family of neuroactive peptides which into rats elicit proconflict responses when injected intraventricularly (i.c.v.) (19,34). In rat brain, the DBI location, structure, and function have been exstensively studied (22). Two major bioactive processing products have been identified: one is DBI fragment 33-50, also termed ODN (octadecaneuropeptide), and the other is DBI framgent 17-50, termed TTN (triakontadecaneuropeptide) (34). These natural processing products of DBI in rat brain act at the allosteric modulatory center of various $GABA_A$ receptor subtypes with different affinities and share with DBI the pharmacological properties of facilitating proconflict behavior when injected icv into rats subjected to the Vogel test. ODN and TTN coexist in neurons with glutamic acid decarboxylase (a marker of GABAergic neurons) and are coreleased with GABA after K^+ or veratridine- induced depolarization (15).

DBI IN NEUROPSYCHOPATHOLOGY

An alteration of GABAergic transmission may play a role in the etiopathogenesis of depression and anxiety disorders such as panic attacks (5,25). The DBI content of spinal fluid is increased in severe cases of depression with high levels of anxiety (4,17), supporting the possibility that spinal fluid measurements of DBI and of its processing products may be useful in monitoring alterations GABAergic transmission in human brain.

DBI is present in the brain of several mammalian species including man (7,10,20,27,28,33). The regional distribution of DBI in postmortem or in biopsic samples of human brain presents strong analogies with DBI observed in rat brain (16,18). The highest concentration of DBI is found in neo-cortical and limbic areas, cerebellum, and brainstem, while the lowest content is found in the basal ganglia. Although the structure of DBI appears to be phylogenetically conserved, the homology is not absolute. In fact, no cross-reactivity is observed between the antisera produced against rat and human DBI . The isolation of cDNA clones has allowed the deduction of amino acid sequences in both rat and human DBI and has revealed that the mRNA for human DBI encodes a peptide of 104 amino acid residues, while the mRNA for rat DBI encodes a peptide of 87 amino acid residues (20). This difference is due to the presence of 60 nucleotides in the

5'end of the human mRNA which are absent in the rat clone. This major difference and other single amino acid mutations in the homologous portion of rat and human DBI may be important determinants for different posttranslational processing of the peptide in rat and human brain.

Since posttranslational processing products of human DBI have not been yet purified and sequenced, we became concerned with procedures for the purification and identification of DBI processing present in human cerebrospinal fluid (CSF) and in human brain.

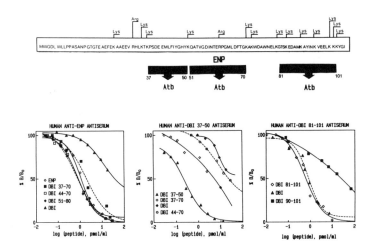

Fig. 1 Top: Primary amino acid structure of human brain DBI and putative cleavage sites at lysine and arginine residues. The filled bars (beneath the primary structure of DBI) indicate the synthetic fragments against which antisera (Atb) were raised in rabbits. Bottom: Cross-reactivity of antisera directed against ENP (DBI 51-70), DBI 37-50, DBI 81-101. Anti-ENP antiserum fails to cross-react with DBI synthetic fragments: 15-30, 17-25, 1-19, 37-50, 30-40, 71-80, 81-101, 90-101. Anti-DBI 37-50 antiserum fails to cross-react with DBI synthetic fragments: 1-19, 15-30, 30-40, ENP, 51-80, 70-80, 81-101, 90-101. Anti-DBI 81-101 antiserum cross-reacts only with DBI 90-101. None of the antisera cross-react with DBI-unrelated poly peptides: physolaemin, neurokinin A, Arg[8]-vasopressin, galanin, NPY, CRF, histone, lysozime, enkephalin, SP, VIP, and CCK.

PROCESSING PRODUCTS OF DBI IN HUMAN BRAIN

a) Quantitative studies

Three different polyclonal antisera were raised against synthetic DBI fragments and were used to identify and characterize the posttranslational processing products of human brain DBI (Fig. 1). The antisera raised in rabbits against human DBI 51-70 (eikosaneuropeptide or ENP), DBI 37-50, and DBI 81-101 were used at a final titer of 5×10^3 and displayed a high degree of affinity and specificity for the respective antigens. Anti-ENP antiserum has an IC_{50} value of 1 nM for ENP (the concentration of ENP giving 50% displacement of label) and exhibits a higher affinity for the synthetic DBI fragments that include the ENP structure (DBI 37-70, 44-70 and 51-80) (Fig.1) . The other synthetic DBI fragments structurally unrelated to ENP fail to be recognized by ENP antiserum, which has an affinity for the entire DBI structure 50-fold lower than that of ENP. The antiserum directed against DBI 37-50 has an IC_{50} value for its antigen of 0.5 nM, while the affinity for DBI is 200-fold lower. The antiserum directed against DBI 37-50 has IC_{50} values for DBI 44-70 and DBI 37-70 of 10 and 50 nM, respectively. The third antiserum used was raised against DBI 81-101. This antiserum has an IC_{50} value for DBI 81-101 of 0.8 nM and cross-reacts with DBI with slightly weaker potency. The fragment DBI 90-101 is recognized by DBI 81-101 antiserum with an IC50 of 16 nM.

To identify the different DBI processing products in human brain, postmortem cerebellum was extracted in hot 1 M acetic acid and the 45.000xg supernatant was fractioned by reverse phase HPLC on a uBondapack C_{18} column. The HPLC fractions were analyzed by using the three antisera described above and an anti-DBI antiserum previously characterized (18). Fig. 2 shows the HPLC separation of the ENP-like immunoreactivity and DBI-like immunoreactivity in postmortem cerebellum. Several peaks of ENP-like immunoreactivity can be recognized. The peak that elutes with the highest percentage of acetonitrile corresponds to DBI. In fact, this peak immunoreacts with anti-DBI antiserum and emerges from the HPLC column with a retention time identical to that of natural DBI. An ENP immunoreactive peak emerging at 29% acetonitrile has a retention time identical to that of the synthetic ENP. SDS-PAGE analysis attributes to this peak a molecular size of approximately 2.4 kDa. On this evidence we have tentatively identified the material associated with this peak as ENP (DBI 51-70). Five other ENP-like immunoreactive peaks indicated in Fig. 2 as a, b, c, d and e can be detected. These peaks were eluted from HPLC with a retention time different from that of the synthetic peptides reported in Fig. 1.

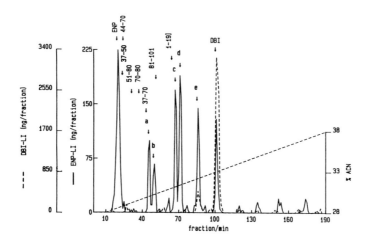

Fig. 2 Reverse-phase HPLC separation of postmortem human cerebellum. Acetic acid extracts were applied onto a uBondapack C_{18} column and chromatographed by using a linear gradient (0-28% in 10 min and 28-38% in 3 hrs; mobile phase= acetonitrile-0.1% TFA; flow rate= ml/min). The fractions were tested with anti-ENP and anti-DBI antisera by radioimmunoassay. The arrows indicate the elution positions of the synthetic fragments.

An immunoreactive profile similar to that obtained with cerebellar extracts (see Fig. 2) is obtained when the cerebrospinal fluid is subjected to HPLC fractionation, suggesting that the peaks present in post mortem cerebellar extracts are not artifacts of a postmortem degradation but rather are natural processing products of DBI. Moreover, an HPLC analysis of the ENP-like immunoreactive peaks in postmortem brain structures (occipital and frontal cortex, hippocampus, thalamus and putamen) reveals that all peaks in the cerebellum and CSF are also present in these brain structures. However, in different brain structures the amount of peptide present in each immunoreactive peak measured as percent of DBI present in each structure is different, suggesting that DBI undergoes regional and cell specific posttranslational processing which gives rise to a specific profile of DBI processing product in each brain structure that we have analyzed.

b) Studies of chemical structures

To acquire information on the amino acid sequences of these peptides, the same HPLC fractions previously quantified with immunochemical procedures using ENP (DBI 51-70) and DBI antisera were analyzed with antisera directed against DBI 37-50 and 81-101. All the HPLC peaks detected with anti ENP antiserum (with the exception of the peak corresponding to ENP) are recognized by anti DBI 37-50 antiserum (Table. 1), whereas only peaks d and e are immunopositive with anti DBI 81-101 antiserum (Table. 1). These observations, taken together with the molecular size of each peak determined by Bio-gel P10 and Western blot analysis, allow tentative predictions of the molecular structure for each ENP immunopositive peaks (Table. 1). Hence, peaks a, b and c that have an apparent molecular size of 3-4 kDa and are recognized by both anti-ENP and anti-DBI 37-50 antisera but not by anti DBI-81-101 antiserum, may include the sequence of DBI 37-70. Peak d with a molecular size of approximately 4 kDa is recognized by the three antisera and may contain the DBI sequence 37-90. Peak e is recognized by the three antisera; however, it has a molecular size of approximately 8 kDa, supporting the inference that it might correspond to DBI 37-101. The exact amino acid sequence of each DBI processing product is presently undergoing a more stringent screening.

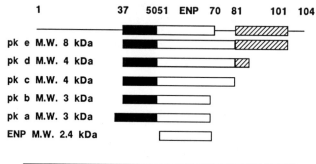

Antisera	ENP	a	b	c	d	e
Anti-DBI	-	-	-	-	-	+/-
Anti-ENP	+	+	+	+	+	+
Anti-DBI 37-50	-	+	+	+	+	+
Anti-DBI 81-101	-	-	-	-	+	+

Table 1. Possible structure of DBI processing products based on the cross-reactivity of the ENP-like peaks (ENP, a, b, c, d and e) with antisera directed against DBI 37-50 (filled bars) and DBI 81-101 (dotted bars). The molecular weights were determined by SDS polyacrylamide gel and Bio-gel P10 filtration.

DBI AND ITS PROCESSING PRODUCTS IN HEPATIC ENCEPHALOPATHY.

The biological significance of the differential processing of the DBI precursor in human CNS remains to be clarified. Although the role of DBI in human brain is not fully understood, there is evidence that the brain steady-state of this peptide might be altered during GABAergic transmission abnormalities. For example, in patients with severe depression with an apparent dysfunction of GABAergic transmission, an increase of CSF DBI content has been reported (4,17). Recently, we have observed that DBI content is elevated 4-fold in the CSF of patients suffering from hepatic encephalopathy (H.E.) (30).
A current theory proposes that the encephalopathy following fulminant hepatic failure is associated with an activation of GABAergic transmission (3,13,14,26). Recently, therapeutic success in the treatment of this disease has been reported using a benzodiazepine antagonist, flumazenil. An alleviation of H.E. symptomatology as well as a concominant improvement in the EEG-graphic alterations has been reported (2,14,21,31,32). Based on this evidence, the existence in this disease of endogenous factors capable of up-regulating GABAergic tone by a positive allosteric modulation including the activation of the benzodiazepine binding sites has been suggested (29,30). Therefore, the levels of DBI and its processing products were analyzed in CSF and in different brain areas of patients with H.E. The DBI content was found to be increased several-fold in the CSF of these patients but it was found to be decreased in cerebellum (Fig. 3) as well as in all the brain areas so far analyzed.
The increase observed in the DBI content of CSF did not correlate with plasma DBI content, suggesting a primary CNS origin of the peptide detected in spinal fluid. The enhancement of CSF DBI content showed a positive correlation with the clinical stages of the disease (30). Moreover, the normalization of awareness observed in two patients subjected to orthotopic liver transplant corresponded with the normalization of CSF DBI content (30). That this increase is specific for H.E. is also revealed by the normal DBI content observed in patients with liver disease not associated with changes in mental status and in patients without H.E. (30). When the DBI posttranslational processing products present in the CSF of these patients were fractioned on reverse phase HPLC, an increased amount of all ENP-like immunoreactive peaks was observed. However, in brain structures of other patients who died with this disease, DBI processing products (peaks ENP, a, b, c, d and e) were decreased. At the present, the data available are limited and it is difficult to conclude that the increase in CSF DBI content observed in these patients derives from an increased utilization of both DBI and its processing products or from an enhanced DBI turnover rate or from both events occurring simultaneously.

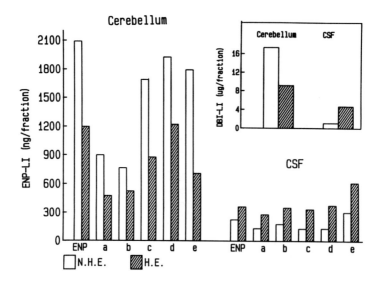

Fig. 3 ENP-LI and DBI-LI (insert) in CSF and in postmortem cerebellum of patients with hepatic encephalopathy (H.E.) and without hepatic encephalopathy (N.H.E.). The cerebellar extract (150mg wet/weight) or CSF (10 ml) were analyzed after reverse-phase HPLC separation as described in the legend of Fig. 2. The results are representative of a single patient. Similar results were obtained in three other patients.

CONCLUSION

In postmortem human brain, six different peptide fragments have been identified as natural posttranslational processing products of DBI. The molecular structure of one of these peptides, ENP, has been inferred by partial sequence analysis, SDS-PAGE, and immunochemistry of HPLC eluates. These analyses contribute evidence suggesting that this peptide is DBI 51-70 (ENP). The exact structure of the other DBI fragments detected in the biological materials studied remains to be determined. Evidence available suggests that the formation of these fragments is not due to non-specific degradation of DBI. Moreover, the results obtained by comparing the immunological properties of these fragments and their molecular size estimated by SDS-PAGE analysis allow the prediction of their approximate structural characteristics. Therefore, peaks a, b and c appear to contain the DBI sequence 37-70, while peaks d and e may include DBI sequences 37-90 and 37-101 respectively.

At present the biological significance of DBI processing products in human brain is not known. However, their uneven distribution in the various brain structures indicates that in human brain differences in posttranslational processing of DBI exist in subpopulations of neurons.

In patients with H.E., DBI processing products and DBI itself are increased in CSF but are decreased in brain. These findings suggest an elevated rate of DBI utilization in HE patients. In addition, an increased synthesis and processing of DBI might also be hypothesized.

All this evidence taken together encourages further work in this area to continue this work. It appears that the study of DBI and of its processing products in cerebrospinal fluid might became a potential marker of brain GABAergic tone.

REFERENCES

1. Alho, H., Costa, E., Ferrero, P., Fujimoto, M., Cosenza-Murfy, D. and Guidotti, A. (1985): Science, 229: 179-182.

2. Bansky, G., Meier, P.J., Zeigler, W.H., Walser, H., Schmid, M. and Huber, M. (1985): Lancet, 1: 1324-1325.

3. Baraldi, M. and Zeneroli, M. (1982): Science, 216: 427-428.

4. Barbaccia, M.L., Costa, E., Ferrero, P., Guidotti, A., Roy, A., Sunderland, T., Pickar, D., Paul, S.M., and Goodwin, F.K. (1986): Arch. Gen. Psychiat., 43: 1143-1147.

5. Bartholin, G., Lloyd, K.G., Morselli, P.L. (1986): GABA and Mood Disorders, Experimental and Clinical Research, Lers, Vol. 4, Raven Press, New York.

6. Bender, A.S. and Hertz, L. (1986): Europ. J. Pharmac., 13: 335-336.

7. Besman, M.J., Yanagibashi, K., Lee, T.D., Kawamura, M., Hall, P.F. and Shively, J.E. (1989): Proc. Natl. Acad. Sci., 86: 4897-4901.

8. Bormann, J., Ferrero, P., Guidotti, A. and Costa, E. (1985): Reg. Peptides, Suppl., 4: 33-45.

9. Bormann, J. (1988): Trends in Neuroscience, 11: 112-116.

10. Chen, Z.W., Agerberth, B., Gell, K., Andersson, M., Mutt, V., Ostenson, C.C., Efendi, S., Barros-Soderling, J., Persson, B. and Jornvall, H. (1988): Europ. J. Biochem., 174 (2): 239-245.

11. Costa, E., Alho, H., Santi, M.R., Ferrero, P., Guidotti, A. (1986): In: Hokfelt, T., Fuxe, K., Pernow, B., eds. Progress in Brain Research, vol 68, Elsevier Science Publ., New York, pp. 343-356.

12. Eipper, B.A., May, V., Cullen, E.I., Sato, S.M., Murthy, A.S. and Mains, R.E. (1987): In: Psychopharmacology: The third generation of progress, Y. Herbert Meltzer, pp. 385-400, Raven Press, New York.

13. Ferenci, P., Grimm, G., Gangle, A. (1987): Hepatology, 7: 1064-1067.

14. Ferenci, P., Schafer, D.F., Kleinberger, G., Hoofnagle, J.H. and Jones, E.A. (1983): Lancet, ii: 811-814.

15. Ferrarese, C., Alho, H., Guidotii, A. and Costa, E. (1987): Neuropharmacology, 26: 1011-1018.

16. Ferrarese, C., Apollonio, I., Frigo, M., Pioliti, R., Tamma, F. and Frattola, L. (1989): Neurology, 39: 443-445.

17. Ferrero, P., Benna, P., Costa, E., Tarenzi, L., Baggio, G., Bergamasco, B. and Bergamini, L. (1988): J. Neurol. Sci., 87: 327-349.

18. Ferrero, P., Costa, E., Conti-Tronconi, B. and Guidotti, A. (1986): Brain Res., 399: 136-142.

19. Ferrero, P., Guidotti, A., Conti-Tronconi, B. and Costa, E. (1984): Neuropharmacology, 23: 1359-1362.

20. Gray, P.W., Glaister, D., Seeburg, P., Guidotti, A. and Costa, E. (1986): Pro. Natl. Acad. Sci., 83: 7547-7551.

21. Grimm, G., Lenz, K., Kleinberger, G., Laggner, A., Druml, W., Schneeweiss, B., Gremmel, F. and Holzner, F. (1987): J.Hepatology, Suppl., 4: S21.

22. Guidotti, A., Forchetti, C.M., Corda, M.G., Konkel, D., Bennett, C.D. and Costa, E. (1983): Proc. Natl. Acad. Sci., 80: 3531-3535.

23. Guidotti, A., Alho, H., Berkovich, A., Cox, D.H., Ferrarese, C., Slobadyansky, E., Santi, M.R. and Costa, E. (1989): In: Allosteric Modulation of Amino Acid Receptors: Therapeutic Implications, E.A. Barnard and E. Costa eds., pp. 109-123, Raven Press, New York.

24. Hokfelt, T., Meister, B., Melander, T., Schalling, M., Staines, W., Millhorn, D., Seroogy, K., Tsuruo, Y., Holets, V., Ceccatelli, S., Villar, M., Ju, G., Freedman, J., Olson, L., Lindh, B., Bartfai, T., Le Greves, P., Terenius, L., Post, C., Mollenholt, P., Dean, J. and Goldestein, M. (1988): In Fidia Research Foundation Neuroscience Award Lectures, Vol.2, pp. 61-113, Raven Press, New York.

25. Hommer, D.W., Skolnick, P., Paul, S.M. (1987): In: Psychopharmacology: The Third Generation of Progress, Ed., H.Y. Meltzer, pp. 977-983 Raven Press, NY.

26. Jones, E.A., Gammal, S.H. (1988): In Arias IM Jakoby W.B., Popper, H. eds., The Liver: Biology and Pathobiology, pp. 985-1005, Raven Press, New York.

27. Marquardt, H., Todaro, G.J. and Shoyab, M. (1986): J. Biol. Chem., 261: 9727-9731.

28. Mocchetti, I., Einstein, R. and Brosius, J. (1986): Proc. Natl. Acad. Sci., 83: 7221-7225.

29. Mullen, K.D., Mendelson, W.B., Martin, J.V. (1988): Lancet, 1: 457-459.

30. Rothstein, J.D., Mekhann, G., Guarneri, P., Barbaccia, M.L., Guidotti, A. and Costa, E. (1989): Ann. Neurol., 26: 57-62.

31. Scollo-Lavizzari, G. (1985): Lancet, 1: 1324 (Letter).

32. Scollo-Lavizzari, G. and Steinmann, E. (1983): Eur. Neurol., 22: 7-11.

33. Shoyab, M., Gentry, L.E., Marquardt, H. and Todaro, G.J. (1986): J. Biol. Chem., 261: 11968-11973.

34. Slobodyansky, E., Guidotti, A., Wambebe, C., Berkovich, A. and Costa, E. (1989): J. Neurochem., 53: 1276-1284.

GABA and Benzodiazepine Receptor Subtypes, edited by Giovanni Biggio and Erminio Costa. Raven Press, New York © 1990.

BENZODIAZEPINE BINDING INHIBITORY ACTIVITY (B.B.I.A.) IN HUMAN PLASMA

D. Marazziti, S. Michelini, *^C. Martini, *G. Giannaccini, G.B. Cassano, and *A. Lucacchini

Department of Psychiatry, via Roma 67, and *"Istituto Policattedra di Discipline Biologiche", via Bonanno 6, University of Pisa, 56100 Pisa, Italy, ^"Istituto di Chimica Biologica", University of Parma, 43100 Parma, Italy.

The current hypothesis on the mode of action of benzodiazepines (BDZ), one of the most widely prescribed drugs, is focused on the interaction with specific binding sites discovered in the brain a decade ago (8, 13). Actually, it is well estabilished that BDZ binding sites are related to, and are part of a supramolecular complex including binding sites for the inhibitory neurotransmitter GABA and a membrane channel permeable to chloride ions where compounds such as picrotoxin and barbiturates may bind. The sites for BDZ seem to be present only on the GABA-A receptor complex consisting of 4 subunits, 2 called beta which are specific for the GABA, and 2 alpha specific for the BDZ (12). The binding of GABA to its site provokes a dramatic increase of the permeability to chloride ions and subsequent hyperpolarization of the neuron (1). The BDZ facilitate the GABA transmission and, although the molecular bases of these events are still unknown, the research in this field has reached considerable results, if compared with other psychotropic drugs. This may be due to the wide prescribtion of BDZ and, even more, to the high incidence of anxiety, and to the efforts towards the biological understanding of this universal disorder. The characterization of the specific binding sites for BDZ gave rise to another approach to the biochemistry of anxiety represented by the search for possible endocoids with agonistic or antagonistic activity on such sites. Among the several proposed compounds, DBI (3), BDZ-like compounds (11), oleic and decosohexenoic acid (9), and n-butyl-beta-carboline (10), are the most recent worthy of mention.

Previously (2, 4) we described a 3H-flunitrazepam (3H-FLU) binding inhibitory activity in deproteinized sera from psychiatric patients, which was lacking in healthy controls, in the range of concentrations used at that time (10-1000 ul). Later (5), this activity was also detected in healthy controls and was called Benzodiazepine Binding Inhibitory Activity (B.B.I.A.). A preliminary biochemical analysis showed the low molecular weight, the heath stability and the resistance to some peptidases of B.B.I.A..

With this research, we provide additional data on the presence of B.B.I.A. in a large group of both psychiatric patients and healthy controls together with further biochemical characteristics.

SUBJECTS AND METHODS

Twenty-five patients (6 males and 19 females; age between 30 and 14, mean+SD: 45.7+13.1) affected by major depression, and 25 patients (13 males and 12 females; age between 18 and 40, mean+SD: 30.8+5.7) affected by panic disorder, according to DSM III-R criteria, recruited at the Psychiatric Department of the University of Pisa, were included. Twelve patients with panic disorder were also suffering from agoraphobia. The controls were 25 healthy volunteers (12 males and 13 females; age between 26 and 41; mean+SD: 28.7+3.1), with no concomitant physical illness as well as familial or past personal history of psychiatric disorders. The patients were drug-free for at least one year and the controls had never taken psychotropic drugs. All the subjects gave their informed consent to the study.

Twelve healthy controls, out of the total of 25, were tested another time 10 min. before sitting for a difficult university exam (the results of this study were object of a previous paper, submitted for publication).

Twenty ml of venous blood were drawn from fasting subjects between 9 and 11 a.m. After serum protein removal by means of ultrafilters (Sep-Pack, C18), the supernatant was assayed on the 3H-FLU binding to bovine brain membranes, prepared as described previously (6). Briefly, bovine brain was homogenized in 10 ml ice-cold 0.32 sucrose for 30 sec. The homogenate was centrifuged at 2,000xg for 5 min at 4°C. The supernatant was centrifuged at 50,000 for 15 min at 4°C. The pellet was osmotically shocked by suspension in 10 volumes of 50 mM Tris-HCl buffer at pH 7.4, and centrifuged at 50,000xg for 15 min at 4°C. Membranes (0.3 mg protein) were incubated with 0.6 nM 3H-FLU in 50 mM Tris-HCl buffer for 45 min at 0°C in the absence (control) and presence of deproteinized sera of the subjects. Incubation was stopped by rapid filtration of the samples through glass-fiber filters washed twice with incubation buffer. Specific binding was obtained in the presence of 0.01 mM diazepam.

The aliquots of serum extracts inhibiting 50% of 3H-FLU (IC50) were determined by log-probit analysis with six to eight concentrations, each performed in triplicate. One inhibitory unit (IU) of B.B.I.A. is defined as the ability of serum to displace 50% of specific 3H-FLU binding in the above assay (one unit corresponds to ∿ 0.9 ng diazepam/ml).

Methanol extract from deproteinized sera was submitted to HPLC on a Beckman Ultrasphere ODS C18 column of 5 um diameter particles 250x4.6 mm i.d., equilibrated with solvent A (15% acetonitrile in 0.1% trifluoroacetic acid). The elution was carried out with a linear gradient from 0 to 45% of solvent B (80% acetonitrile in 0.1% trifluoroacetic acid) over 40 min, at flow rate of 1 ml/min. The absorbance at 230 nm of the eluate was recorded at 0.05 absorbance units at full scale. Aliquots of the fractions eluted from the HPLC column were assayed for their ability to displace the 3H-FLU binding to bovine cortical membranes.

Statistical analyses among the different groups included was assessed by ANOVA one-way analysis of variance, followed by unpaired Student's t-test. The difference between the IU of B.B.I.A. in stressful and calm situation was assessed by paired Student's t-test.

RESULTS

The inhibitory activity (B.B.I.A.) on the 3H-FLU binding to bovine brain membranes was present in all subjects (table 1). It was competitive and reversible (data not shown).

The IU ranged between 333 and 0.1 (mean$\pm$SD: 52.36$\pm$77.62) in the depressed patients, and between 500 and 0.4 (mean$\pm$SD:49.83$\pm$118.06) in the patients affected by panic disorder, with no statistically significant difference between the 2 groups.

The IU ranged between 1.25 and 0.1 (mean$\pm$SD:0.46$\pm$0.28) in the healthy controls sampled in calm situation, significantly lower as compared with the IU of psychiatric patients (p<0.0001). In the 12 subjects sampled immediately before a difficult university exam, the IU increased significantly (mean$\pm$SD:1.05$\pm$3.29) (p<0.004), although the values were still significantly lower than in the patients (p<0.0001).

HPLC column experiments showed the presence of 3 peaks of inhibitory activity (fig. 1) determined by the displacement of the 3H-FLU to bovine brain membranes. The active material obtained from healthy volunteers and patients eluted with the same retention time in the C18 column.

TABLE 1. B.B.I.A. inhibitory unit values of patients and controls

	D	PD	HV
Age	45.7	30.8	28.7
	13.1	5.7	3.1
IU	52.4	49.8	0.46
	77.6	118.06	0.28

D= depressed patients
PD= patients affected by panic disorder
HV= healthy volunteers
Age= years (mean±SD)
IU= inhibitory units (mean±SD)

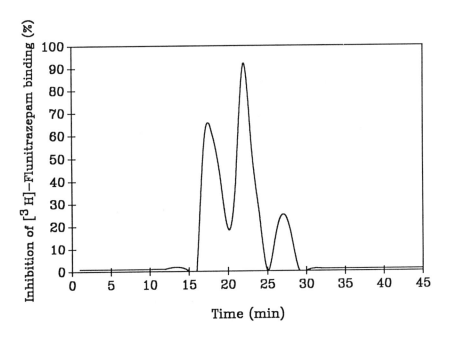

FIG. 1, HPLC of the methanol extract from deproteinized patient sera

DISCUSSION AND CONCLUSIONS

The results of this research show that a plasmatic 3H-FLU binding inhibitory activity (B.B.I.A.) is present in a large group of both psychiatric patients and healthy controls. Psychiatric diagnosis seems not to affect the concentration of B.B.I.A., since no significant difference between depressed and panic disorder patients has been detected. On the contrary, psychiatric patients differ significantly from the healthy controls, being B.B.I.A. higher in the first group.

Our data also indicate that B.B.I.A. levels are subjected to changes in healthy controls undergone stressful situation, such as that of sitting for an university exam. In this case B.B.I.A. concentrations increased significantly, although they didn't reach the values found in the patients.

Preliminary results on healthy subjects undergone physical stress are in agreement with the present report (data not shown). This is the first demonstration of stress-related changes of a possible endocoid for BDZ receptors, in humans. Previously, Medina et al. (7) have reported an increase in the brain n-butyl-beta-carboline in rats and how this could be reversed by diazepam.

On the basis of our researches, it is conceivable to hypothesize a role of B.B.I.A. in the pathophysiology of both physiological and pathological anxiety, being the difference between the 2 kinds of anxiety only quantitative.

A preliminary biochemical analysis of B.B.I.A. has shown that it is dialyzable, heat-stable, insensitive to proteolytic degradation or to treatment with strong acids. B.B.I.A. is specific for BDZ central receptor which binds with high affinity (below nM), compatible with "in vivo" interactions. No activity has been detected on the binding of 3H-Ro5-4864 (specific for the peripheral BDZ receptor), on the binding of 3H-muscimol, and on the binding of 3H-SCH 23390, specific for the dopamine 1 receptor (5).

HPLC analysis has revealed the presence of 3 peaks of inhibition in both patients and healthy controls eluting with the same retention time.

Analysis of the peaks by mass-fragmentography is in progress.

Acknowledgement. This research was supported by a grant of the italian Ministry of Public Education. S.M. is recipient of a grant of the "A. Buzzati-Traverso" Foundation.

REFERENCES

1. Gallager, D.W., and Tallman, J.F. (1983): Neuropharmacol. 22:1943-1949.

2. Giannaccini, G., Marazziti, D., Martini, C., Pietrini, P., Placidi, G.F., and Lucacchini, A. (1986): Proceedings of the 18th ENA congress, Praha.

3. Guidotti, A., Forchetti, C.M. , Corda, M.G. , Konkel, D., Bennet, C.D., and Costa, E. (1983): Proc. natl. Acad. Sci. USA 80:3531-3535.

4. Marazziti, D., Pietrini, P., Martini, C., Giannaccini, G., Perugi, G., Placidi, G.F., Cassano, G.B., and Lucacchini, A. (1988): Neuropsychobiol. 18:74-76.

5. Marazziti, D., Michelini, S., Martini, C., Giannaccini G., Lucacchini, A., and Cassano, G.B.: Neuropsychobiology (in press).

6. Martini, C., Rigacci, T., and Lucacchini, A. (1983): J. Neurochem. 41:1183-1185.

7. Medina, J.H., Pena, C., Novas, N.L., Paladini, A.C., and De Robertis, E. (1987): Neurochem. Int. 11:255-259.

8. Mohler, H., and Okada, T. (1977): Science192:849-851.

9. Nielsen, M., Witt, M.R., and Thorgensen, H. (1988): Eur. J. Pharmacol. 146:349-353.

10. Pena, C., Medina, J.H., Novas, M.L., Paladini, A.C., and De Robertis, E. (1986): Proc. natl. Acad. Sci. USA 83:4952-4956.

11. Sangameswaran, N.L., Fales, H.M., Friedrich, P., and De Blas, A.L. (1986): Proc. natl. Acad. Sci. USA 83:9236-9240.

12. Schofield, P.R., Darlison, M.G., Fujita, N., Stephenson, F.A., Rodriguez, H., Rhee, L.M., Ramachandran, J., Reale, V., Glencorse, T.A., Seeburg, P., Barnard, E. (1987): Nature, 328:221-227.

13. Squires, R.S. and Braestrup C. (1977): Nature 266 732-737.

GABA and Benzodiazepine Receptor Subtypes,
edited by Giovanni Biggio and Erminio Costa.
Raven Press, New York © 1990.

"SPARE RECEPTORS" AND "PARTIAL AGONISTS" --
ROMANTIC TERMS TO EXPLAIN A PHARMACOLOGY DERIVING FROM THE
STRUCTURAL DIVERSITY OF GABA$_A$ RECEPTORS.

E. Costa

FIDIA-Georgetown Institute for the Neurosciences
Georgetown University Medical School
3900 Reservoir Road, N.W.
Washington, D.C.   20007

Eccles' interpretation (11) of Dale's proposition (10) --
that the transmitter's structural and metabolic profile is
constant in a given class of neurons -- generated the belief
that a neuron synthesizes, stores and releases one and only one
transmitter (11).   Moreover, a relative structural uniformity
of transmitter receptors was deduced from the predictable
pattern of agonist responsiveness of primary transmitter
recognition sites.   This simplistic view of synaptic
transmission persisted for years, until it was shown that
various synaptic signals can coexist in the same neuron (21).
In addition, the amino acid sequence of transmitter receptors
obtained by molecular cloning began to indicate an unsuspected
structural diversity of synaptic GABA$_A$ receptors (22).   Now,
polytypic signalling in synaptic transmission and structural
diversity of receptors are considered an important source of
structural diversity that, in part, explains individual
variability in higher brain functions (6).   Finally, the
evidence that ion channels and enzymes can function as
effectors in synaptic transmission has suggested that synaptic
receptors can be classified as ionotropic (using ion channels),
metabolotropic (using enzymes that generate second messengers),
or mixed function (using second messengers to gate ion
channels).   Along these lines, GABAergic transmission was shown
to include ionotropic GABA$_A$ receptors with muscimol as the
specific agonist and metabolotropic GABA$_B$ receptors with
baclofen as the specific agonist (12,17).   Soon, evidence
emerged supporting the possibility that GABA$_B$ metabolotropic
receptors could operate as mixed function receptors by gating
ion channels via second messengers (1).   The analysis of the

221

dynamic properties of GABA$_A$ and GABA$_B$ receptors, through the construction of transmitter recognition site saturation isotherms occurred with high affinity radioligand binding assay. By comparing binding characteristics of ligands endowed with agonist or antagonist activity to their maximal receptor function modification, it became clear that the latter could be expressed before reaching ligand saturation of transmitter recognition sites. This discrepancy was explained with the descriptive term "spare receptors", thereby defining, in a given tissue, the existence of a pool of transmitter recognition sites uncoupled to the effector system of the receptor under study and, therefore, incapable of eliciting a functional modification. With the adoption of such terminology, it was tacitly assumed that tissues contain a reserve pool of recognition sites ready to compensate for a functional deficit due to lack of available receptors. For instance, before knowing that GABA$_B$ receptors existed, the excess binding of GABA to receptor recognition sites would have been considered to occur at "spare receptors". The presence in a brain structure of a transmitter recognition site pool that is not coupled to an effector may reflect a dynamic equilibrium between the biosynthesis, utilization, and degradation of these sites. Thus, such a dynamic pool may express regulation of transmitter receptor density associated with functional diversity, e.g., shifts in receptor density associated with sub- and supersensitivity of transmitter receptors. However, one cannot and should not dismiss the possibility that GABA$_A$ or GABA$_B$ receptor structural and functional diversity may, in part, explain the discrepancy between the number of binding sites occupied by a given ligand and the number of sites needed to elicit the maximal receptor-mediated modification of a specific function. In the face of present evidence on the structural diversity of transmitter recognition sites coupled with various effectors, the term "spare receptor" cannot be freely used. Before using it one must be sure that there is not present in the tissue a population of transmitter recognition sites coupled to an effector system whose function is not revealed in the functional response monitored.

When the structure-activity relationship was studied for a series of chemically related GABA$_A$ receptor ligands, it was found that various molecules, in the face of an equal saturation of available binding sites, could express various levels of efficacy (16). To explain this further discrepancy, the term "partial agonist" has been used (16). Again, based on the assumption of a structural and functional uniformity of receptors, this term tacitly indicates that only the chemical structural diversity of the molecules under study determined the variability observed in their efficacy. The latter has been related to the specific intrinsic activity of molecules tested, and, a priori, participation of a receptor structure diversity was excluded. Also, this nomenclature was romantically devised to defend a given assumption, without considering the dangers of hiding differences in response quality or quantity due to molecular specificity of receptor subtypes.

Structural diversity of GABA_A receptors: role of the allosteric modulatory centers

Early studies of the mode of action of anxiolytic benzodiazepines have indicated that their pharmacological profile could be explained by action on an allosteric modulatory center conceived as a receptor regulatory mechanism detected first in GABA_A receptors (7,9). It was proposed that benzodiazepines modulate the probability of receptor responsiveness to GABA by changing the kinetic interaction between the primary transmitter and its recognition sites (7). This suggestion has been supported by the finding that benzodiazepines are inactive in the absence of GABA; when GABA is present, however, they increase its efficacy, probably by facilitating the formation or persistence of the the bi-liganded stage of receptor-ligand interaction (4). In kinetic terms, the maximal efficacy of GABA action is not increased by benzodiazepines, but maximal levels of efficacy are reached with GABA concentrations lower than those required to elicit maximal responses in the absence of these anxiolytics (28).

Supporting this suggestion is the finding that channel open time, or other kinetic parameters of single channel dynamics, are not changed by benzodiazepines (4); however, channel bursting activity (24) is greatly enhanced by these drugs (4). The result is an increase of total ion current over time that can explain the potentiation of GABA action. Moreover, GABA receptor down regulation occurring in particular experimental conditions is facilitated by benzodiazepines (2). In the face of this mechanism of action (6), the terminology "partial agonist" (16) cannot be used to describe the intrinsic activity of drugs acting as positive or negative allosteric modulators of transmitter receptors (6). In fact, this action depends on the availability of the endogenous agonist and consists of a facilitation of the channel bursting activity, presumably produced by persistence of the biliganded form of the receptor. Moreover, benzodiazepines not only facilitate GABA action but also facilitate the desensitization of GABA receptors (2), probably because they increase the time of interaction between GABA and its receptors. When high doses of benzodiazepines are used, the facilitation can lead to a quick desensitization of GABA operated channel gating. The use of the term "agonist" (16) to classify drugs that are devoid of agonistic activity "per se", but modulate the action of GABA released from nerve terminals through physiological mechanisms, should be questioned.

By using the term partial agonist (16), the revolutionary concept brought into pharmacology by the potentiation of transmitter   action   with   benzodiazepines,   due   to   a   better transmitter-targetting   following   drug   action   on   the   modulatory centers   of   the   GABA   receptors,   is   hidden   (16).   This   positive modulation   cannot   be   considered   agonistic   because   it   is   not expressed   when   the   concentration   of   GABA   present   evokes   maximal responses,   or   when   GABA   is   not   present.   In   fact,   this   action is   different   from   the   potentiation   of   a   transmitter   response   by uptake   blockers   because,   unlike   uptake   blockers,   it   varies according   to   the   structural   diversity   of   the   modulatory   center present   in   a   given $GABA_A$ receptor   subtype   (6,14).

Positive and Negative Modulation of $GABA_A$ Receptors

While   complete   agreement   has   been   reached   on   the   GABAergic mediation   of   benzodiazepine   action   (6),   the   interpretation   of the   physiological   significance   of   the   allosteric   modulatory center,   where   benzodiazepines   act   (6),   is   still   a   matter   of controversy   (16).   One   group   (7)   believes   that   benzodiazepines act   on   an   allosteric   modulatory   center   that   has   an   intrinsic regulatory   function   on   the   physiological   operation   of   the   GABA gated Cl^- channels   (6).   Supporting   evidence   shows   that   there is   an   endogenous   peptide,   isolated   and   purified   from   brain extracts   by   monitoring   their   ability   to   displace   diazepam (Diazepam   Binding   Inhibitor   =   DBI),   which   is   stored   and synthesized   in   neurons   of   rats,   human,   and   bovine   brain (8,13,19).   DBI   functions   as   the   precursor   for   biologically active   peptides   which   selectively   act   as   negative   allosteric modulators   of   specific $GABA_A$ receptor   subtypes   (14).   Another benzodiazepine   derivative,   flumazenil,   acts   isosterically   on the   recognition   sites   for   anxiolytic   benzodiazepines,   but   it   is devoid   of   intrinsic   activity   on   the   allosteric   modulatory center   regulating   the   efficacy   of   GABA   in   gating Cl^- channels (15).   Flumazenil,   by   virtue   of   its   high   affinity   binding   to the   allosteric   modulatory   center,   prevents   the   action   of   other ligands   on   the $GABA_A$ receptor   modulatory   center.   This   drug antagonizes   both   anxiolytic   benzodiazepines,   endowed   with positive   modulatory   action,   and   anxiogenic β-carbolines, endowed   with   negative   modulatory   action   (29)   on $GABA_A$ operation.

There   is   evidence   that   different   GABAergic   neurons   have different   types   of   allosteric   modulatory   centers;   for   instance, those   in   the   spinal   cord   neurons   lack   binding   capacity   for β-carboline   derivatives   (25).

Another   group   of   investigators   (16)   departs   from   this physiologically   slanted   interpretation   of   benzodiazepine   action and   assumes   that   the   high   affinity   binding   site   for benzodiazepine   and β-carboline   derivatives   is   devoid   of physiological   significance   and   represents   exclusively   a structural   detail   in   the   configuration   of   the $GABA_A$ receptor where   anxiolytic   benzodiazepines,   anxiogenic β-carbolines, and   flumazenil   happen   to   bind.   This   group   of   investigators believes   that   various   benzodiazepines   act   as   agonists   with   full or partial efficacy.

Recent findings on the structure of $GABA_A$ receptors indicate that they are hetero-oligomeric channels (27) comprising four subunits (26). The α, β, (26) and γ (22) subunits have been cloned from brain cDNA libraries and their amino acid sequences have been derived (26). These studies have indicated that both bovine and human brain express several molecular forms of each subunit (22). This raises the possibility of a high degree of $GABA_A$ receptor diversity due to the assembly of various molecular forms of the subunits in forming various configurations of $GABA_A$ receptors. It is important that a frequent site for the expression of $GABA_A$ receptor subunit diversity is located in the extracellular receptor domain (22,26); probably the allosteric modulatory center and the GABA recognition site of the $GABA_A$ receptor are also located here . Thus, it would not seem impossible that the allosteric modulatory center, which is a structural site responsible for functional receptor diversity, might have physiological significance. Moreover, such a functional possibility receives futher support because it is located with a receptor site expressing structural diversity of $GABA_A$ receptors.

The assembly in expression vectors of various cDNAs encoding for different molecular forms of $GABA_A$ receptor subunits has allowed transfection and expression of various molecular forms of $GABA_A$ receptors in neuronal cell lines devoid of such receptors, or in Xenopus laevis oocytes. The function of these artificially assembled GABA regulated Cl⁻ channels has been studied. This work has so far indicated (3,18,22,23): 1) cell transfection with cDNA $\alpha+\beta$, only α, and only β subunits leads to the expression of Cl⁻ channels that can be operated with GABA; this action can be inhibited by picrotoxin and greatly facilitated with barbiturates, but not with benzodiazepines; in such transfected receptors the channel opening inhibition with β-carboline derivatives is also lacking; 2) expression of the full capacity of benzodiazepine positive modulation or of β-carboline negative modulation requires that the γ_2 subunit be present; 3) the assembly of various subunits is associated with variability in GABA potency and with varying degrees of desensitization susceptibility to GABA channel gating; and 4) the $GABA_A$ receptor present in astrocyte membranes may have a peculiarly structured allosteric center because these receptors appear to allow β-carboline to increase the probability of GABA action (5). Hence, β-carbolines cannot elicit a negative modulation of astrocyte $GABA_A$ receptors but can cause a positive modulation similar to that elicited by anxiolytic benzodiazepines (5).

If all these data are considered, it appears that the site of action of benzodiazepines should be viewed as a functional entity of $GABA_A$ receptors, now open to the investigation of its physiological role. Moreover, the structural diversity of this site suggests that some classes of benzodiazepines may act preferentially on specific structural profiles of GABA$_A$ receptors. By virtue of this selectivity, the possibility of obtaining new benzodiazepine classes with pharmacological profiles and therapeutic indications different from those of diazepam might be envisioned.

Can the "partial agonist" action of certain benzodiazepines be due to the structural diversity of GABA$_A$ receptors?

As an example of the molecular mechanisms that might explain the partial agonist action of benzodiazpines, we would like to compare the high affinity binding and maximal anticonvulsant action of clonazepam and diazepam (Table 1).

TABLE 1: High affinity binding (B$_{max}$) and maximal bicuculline antagonism by clonazepam and diazepam in rats.

Benzodiazepine	Bicuculline* μmole/rat/i.v.	B$_{max}$ (nM)				
		OB	C	CB	ST	SC
Clonazepam	0.78	2.3	2.2	2.1	0.9	n.d.
Diazepam	1.3	2.2	2.0	1.8	1.6	0.90

OB: Olfactory Bulb; C: Cortex; CB: Cerebellum; ST: Striatum; SP: Spinal Cord; n.d.: non-detectable;
* Diazepam doses from (5 to 10 μmole/kg i.v.) - Clonazepam doses (from 0.35 to 2 μmole/kg i.v.).
From Ph.D. dissertation in pharmacology by J. Schlichting (Georgetown University , Washington, D.C.)

The maximal dose of bicuculline antagonized by 5 or 10 μmole/kg i.v. of diazepam is 1.3 μmole/rat i.v.; in contrast, 0.3 or 2 μmole/kg i.v. of clonazepam can antagonize only 0.78 μmole/rat i.v. of bicuculline. This difference in efficacy of the two drugs occurr even though the binding affinity of the two drugs to brain membranes is similar (Table 1). Using the romantic terminology discussed earlier, one could say that diazepam counteracts the action of bicuculline as a full agonist while clonazepam does so as a partial agonist. This nomenclature explains the difference in efficacy by attributing an intrinsic activity to clonazepam lower than that of diazepam. However, if one keeps in mind GABA$_A$ receptor diversity, it can be surmised that the GABA$_A$ receptor modulatory action of diazepam is more generalized than that of clonazepam. In other words, clonazepam fails to act on one or more subtypes of those GABA$_A$ receptors modulated by diazepam. To evaluate this hypothesis, we studied the high affinity binding of the two drugs to various brain structures and concluded that, indeed, the two drugs bind to a similar population of receptors in membranes prepared from olfactory bulbs, cortex, and cerebellum. Thus, on the basis of these results, one might conclude that the anticonvulsant action of clonazepam could be defined using the romantic term "partial antagonist" (Table 1). However, if one considers the specific binding of the two drugs on the receptor in striatum and spinal cord membranes, it could be inferred that the binding specificity displayed by diazepam and clonazepam for the various molecular forms of the GABA$_A$ receptor is different. Perhaps the different efficacies of the two drugs as antagonists of bicuculline, an isosteric GABA$_A$ recognition site blocker, could be due to the lack of action of clonazepam on the modulatory center of rat spinal cord, a structure rich in GABA$_A$ receptors susceptible to the bicuculline blockade. To test the hypothesis that GABA$_A$ receptor diversity is the source for the partial antagonistic action of clonazepam, the high affinity binding profile of various benzodiazepines was tested in cerebellar and spinal cord membranes. These data are reported in Table 2.

TABLE 2: K_D and B_{max} of ^{3}H-diazepam, ^{3}H-flumazenil, ^{3}H-clona-zepam, ^{3}H-zolpidem, and ^{3}H-DMCM binding to membranes prepared from rat cerebellum and spinal cord.

Benzodiazepine	Cerebellum		Spinal Cord (nM)	
	K_D*	B_{max}*	K_D*	B_{max}*
^{3}H-diazepam	1.5	1.8	1.7	0.90
^{3}H-flumazenil	1.0	1.8	3.0	0.85
^{3}H-clonazepam	1.5	2.1	n.d.	n.d.
^{3}H-zolpidem	7.0	1.3	n.d.	n.d.
^{3}H-DMCM	5.0	1.8	n.d.	n.d.

* K_D=nM; B_{max}=pmol/mg protein
n.d.: non-detectable
(Massotti, M., Memo, M., Schlichting, J. This laboratory, unpublished)

It is clear from these data that the binding profiles of spinal cord membranes differ from those of cerebellum, and this is presumably due to the different subtype of GABA$_A$ receptor present in this structure. Interestingly enough, receptor diversity can be evidenced by the different properties of a number of ligands in binding to the allosteric modulatory centers of cerebellum and spinal cord (Table 2).

Conclusion:

The data and the arguments presented tend to support the hypothesis that the allosteric modulatory center is an important source of functional diversity that may be associated with structural diversity of GABA$_A$ receptors. This encourages further studies of both the physiological significance of GABA$_A$ receptor structural diversity vis-a-vis the functional role associated with this diversity and the modulatory center qualitative functional diversity associated with structural diversities. From such studies it may emerge that structure-activity relationship studies of various benzodiazepines, using tests that differentiate various GABA$_A$ receptor subtype functions, may reveal a new classification of these drugs in terms of specificity of action on the allosteric modulatory centers of various GABA$_A$ receptor subtypes. If this is the case, it will be clear that the term "partial agonist" or "partial antagonist" does not apply to drugs acting on structurally variable sites located in specific subtypes of GABA$_A$ receptors. It is my opinion that the pharmacology of the allosteric modulatory centers of GABA$_A$ receptors should not be complicated and confused by the use of romantic descriptive terms that ignore the structural diversity of GABA receptors. It is becoming important to follow this directive in order to develop the pharmacology of benzodiazepines along the new needs resulting from the application of molecular biological techniques to the study of GABA receptors.

REFERENCES

1. Andrade, R., Malenka, R.C. and Nicoll, R.A. (1986): Science, 234: 1261-1263.
2. Biggio, G., Giorgi, O., Concas, A. and Corda, M.G. (1989): In: Allosteric Modulation of Amino Acid Receptors: Therapeutic Implications, edited by E.A. Barnard and E. Costa. pp. 71-89. Raven Press, New York.
3. Blair, L.A.C., Levitan, E.S., Marshall, J., Dionne, V.E. and Barnard, E.A. (1988): Science, 242: 577-579.
4. Bormann, J. and Clapham, D.E. (1985): Proc. Natl. Acad. Sci. USA, 82: 2168-2172.
5. Bormann, J. and Kettenmann, H. (1988): Proc. Natl. Acad. Sci. USA, 85: 9336-9340.
6. Costa, E., Alho, H., Favaron, M. and Manev, H. (1989): In:

Allosteric Modulation of Amino Acid Receptors: Therapeutic Implications, edited by E.A. Barnard and E. Costa. pp. 3-18. Raven Press, New York.

7. Costa, E. and Guidotti, A. (1979): Ann. Rev. Pharmacol. Toxicol., 19: 531-545.

8. Costa, E. and Guidotti, A. (1987): In: Psychopharmacology: The Third Generation of Progress, edited by H.Y. Metzer. pp. 425-435. Raven Press, New York.

9. Costa, E., Guidotti, A., Mao, C. and Suria, A. (1975): Life Science, 17: 167-186.

10. Dale, H.H. (1952): Transmission of Effects from Nerve Endings. Oxford Press, London.

11. Eccles, J.C. (1957): In: The Physiology of Nerve Cells. p. 212. Johns Hopkins Press, Baltimore.

12. Enna, S.J (1983): In: The GABA receptors, edited by S.J. Enna. pp. 1-23. Humana Press, Clifton, New Jersey.

13. Ferrero, P., Santi, M.R., Conti-Tronconi, B., Costa, E. and Guidotti, A. (1986): Brain Res., 399: 136-142.

14. Guidotti, A., Alho, H., Berkovich, A., Cox, D.H., Ferrarese, C., Slobodyansky, E., Santi, M.R. and Wambebe, C. (1989): In: Allosteric Modulation of Amino Acid Receptors: Therapeutic Implications, edited by E.A. Barnard and E. Costa. pp. 109-123. Raven Press, New York.

15. Haefely, W. (1983): In: Benzodiazepine Recognition Site Ligands: Biochemistry and Pharmacology, edited by G. Biggio and E. Costa. pp. 73-93. Raven Press, New York.

16. Haefely, W. (1989): In : Allosteric Modulation of Amino Acid Receptors: Therapeutic Implications, edited by E.A. Barnard and E. Costa. pp. 47-69. Raven Press, New York.

17. Hill, D.R. and Bowery, N.G.: Nature, 290: 149-152.

18. Levitan, E.S., Schofield, P.R., Burt, D.R., Rhee, L.M., Wisden, W., Khler, M., Fujita, N., Rodriguez, H.F., Stephenson, A., Darlison, M.G., Barnard E.A. and Seeburg, P.H. (1988): Nature, 335: 76-79.

19. Marquardt, H., Todero, G.J. and Shoyab, M. (1986): J. Biol. Chem., 261: 9729-9731.

20. McGeer, P.L., Eccles, J.C. and McGeer, E.G. (1978): Molecular Neurobiology and the Mammalian Brain. Plenum Press, New York.

21. Potter, D.D., Furshpan, E.J. and Landis, S.C. (1981): Neurosc. Commentaries, 1: 1-9, 1981.

22. Pritchett, D.B., Sontheimer, H., Shivers, B.D., Ymer, S., Kettenmann, H, Schofield, P.R. and Seeburg, P.H. (1989): Nature, 338: 582-585.

23. Puia, G., Santi, M.R., Vicini, S., Pritchett, D.B., Seeburg, P.H. and Costa, E. (1989, in press): Proc. Natl. Acad. Sci. USA.

24. Sakmann, B., Hamill, O.P. and Bormann, J. (1983): J. Neurol. Transm., 18: 83-95.

25. Santi, M.R., Cox, D.H. and Guidotti, A. (1988): J. Neurochem., 50: 1080-1086.
26. Schofield, P.R., Darlison, M.G., Fujita, N., Burt, D.R., Stephenson, F.A., Rodriguez, H., Rhee, L.M., Ramachandran, J., Rede, B., Glencorse, T.A., Seeburg, P.H. and Barnard, E.A. (1987): Nature, 328: 221-227.
27. Stephenson, F.A. (1988): Biochem. J., 249: 21-32.
28. Study, R. and Barker, J.L. (1981): Proc. Natl. Acad. Sci. USA, 78: 7180-7184.
29. Vicini, S., Mienville, J.M. and Costa, E. (1987): J. Pharm. Exp. Ther., 243:1195-1201.

GABA and Benzodiazepine Receptor Subtypes, edited by Giovanni Biggio and Erminio Costa. Raven Press, New York © 1990.

CONCLUDING REMARKS

Willy Haefely

F.Hoffmann-La Roche Ltd,
Pharmaceutical Research Department
CH-4002 Basel (Switzerland)

The symposium on $GABA_A$/BZ receptor subtypes dealt with the two major areas of ongoing research, namely 1) the structural heterogeneity of this class of receptor-operated anion channels and its possible impact on discrete functional differences between receptor variants and 2) the allosteric modulation of the receptor-channel function by the BZR.

At the last Capo Boi meeting the molecular cloning and sequencing of the predicted α- and ß-subunits of the bovine brain $GABA_A$ receptor was reported (1,8). The heterologous coexpression of the two cRNAs in Xenopus oocytes was reported to direct the synthesis and membrane incorporation of a fully functional $GABA_A$ receptor as shown by the bicuculline-sensitive activation of chloride conductance by GABA and its modulation by a barbiturate and a BZ. This apparently simple situation was to be corrected soon. Now three groups (Seeburg et al.; Möhler et al.; Olsen et al., this symposium) presented evidence for the existence in 3 species of at least 6 α-subunit variants, at least 3 ß-subunit variants and probably of additional γ and ε subunits. Controversial results are being obtained in the electrophysiological study of receptors expressed after injection into oocytes and mammalian cells of various combinations of subunit variants, in particular with respect to allosteric modulation by BZR ligands (11). An initially underestimated methodological problem is being recognized, namely the variable responses to GABA within one experiment, and the complication induced by the $GABA_A$ receptor desensitization occurring with the usually rather long-lasting GABA pulses applied. It is, therefore, impossible at present to state with any certainty how receptor complexes with differing subunit composition differ from each other in GABA affinity, channel conductances and kinetics as well as by the sensitivity to and the direction of modulation by various BZR ligands. $GABA_A$ receptors have been unambiguously shown to exist on neurons, glial cells and adrenal medullary cells. Do distinct cell types express only one specific subset of receptor-channel complexes or a mixture of them? Does a given phenotypic repertoire of $GABA_A$ receptor subtypes relate to functional specialization and to differential sensitivity to drugs acting as allosteric modulators? An intriguing objective of future investigations is the identification of the subunit composition of these various native receptor-channel complexes. Variants of these may mediate differing responses to GABA with respect to sensitivity, amplitude of chloride flux, and desensitization. Of greater interest for pharmacologists is the possible impact of subunit composition on the activity of allosteric modulators of the $GABA_A$ receptors, in particular those acting on the BZR. Are there $GABA_A$ receptors without the modulatory BZR?

Are BZR exclusively located on α-subunits? Do the α-subunit variants and the receptor-channel variants (subtypes) differentially recognize various BZR ligands and differentially transduce their message?

A subclassification of BZRs was proposed already ten years ago (9) based on the preferential affinity of some non-BZ ligands (ß-carbolines, triazolopyridazines) for BZRs in some regions of the CNS. The BZ_1 and BZ_2 receptor concept attempted to account for real or hypothetical differences in the pharmacological profiles of various BZR ligands - unconvincingly, to say the least. This is also illustrated by the more recent proposal (Langer et al., this symposium) that two imidazopyridines produced their effects by preferential action on the BZ_1 subtype. One of these, zolpidem, is reported to have specific hypnotic activity, whereas the other, alpidem, is described as a non-sedative, anxioselective BZR ligand. Obviously, this difference cannot be explained by a BZ_1 subtype preference. Our own unpublished results indicate that zolpidem behaves very much like a conventional full agonist of BZR, whereas alpidem is a partial agonist with very weak intrinsic efficacy; it antagonizes various effects of diazepam very efficiently and has only a borderline anticonflict effect in rats even after very high oral doses (in addition, the very weak potency in vivo as opposed to a high in vitro affinity for the BZR suggests a bioavailability problem).

The structural complexity of $GABA_A$-BZ receptors will necessitate a classification of native receptor variants. As discussed recently with respect to subtypes of 5-HT receptors (6) such a classification should be based primarily on molecular structure. Thus, the classification of BZRs proposed by Langer (7) is rather a step backwards (marketing people may argue differently). Merely replacing the term BZ by omega does not make sense scientifically because the so-called peripheral (or mitochondrial) BZ binding site (Krueger et al., this symposium; 10) and the BZRs that are an integral part of the $GABA_A$ receptor have nothing in common in terms of structure and function and should by no means be classified together in one family. The present state of knowledge and the impending resolution of still open issues suggest that within the next few years a classification can be found that satisfies scientific stringency as well as the need for terms serving as hints to the function. Such a classification may start with the term $GABA_A$ (indicating the GABA-responsive receptor coupled to the anion channel). The various $GABA_A$ receptor subtypes (differing in subunit composition) may be termed $GABA_{A1}$ to $GABA_{Ax}$. The allosteric modulatory receptors on the $GABA_A$ receptor/channel complex may be indicated by a Greek letter, e.g. the BZR by α, the barbiturate receptor by ß and so forth. Subtypes of BZRs could be indicated by an additional number, e.g. the BZ_1 and BZ_2 receptors (if confirmed) could become $GABA_{A\ x\ \alpha 1}$-R and $GABA_{A\ x\ \alpha 2}$-R, respectively.

All macromolecules acting as receptors, i.e. macromolecules containing domains that recognize and bind specifically endogenous signal molecules or exogenous drugs to respond with a conformational change (or a change in charge distribution), are known (or will be found one day) to interact with both agonists and antagonists. This is the core principle of pharmacology. The differing consequences of receptor interaction with agonists and antagonists are due to an intrinsic property of the ligand called intrinsic efficacy, although this property cannot yet be clearly identified in terms of physicochemical properties. It is also commonplace knowledge that intrinsic efficacies between the maximal one (of full agonists) and zero (of pure competitive antagonists) give rise to partial (low efficacy) agonists. The overall pharmacological profile of partial agonist can differ considerably from that of full agonists when submaximal intrinsic efficacy of a ligand combines with differing cell and tissue factors, such as receptor density. BZR ligands show exactly the same behavior at their receptor as ligands (agonists, partial agonists, antagonists) of any other receptor, as shown in a great number of studies on tissues or single cells and in whole animals (as illustrated by Jensen, this symposium). It is, therefore, very logical to apply the same terminology to BZR ligands and to call BZR agonists those ligands that induce a positive allosteric modulation of the $GABA_A$ receptor-mediated chloride channel gating, i.e. enhance or facilitate the action of GABA. As with every other receptor, those ligands of the BZR which fail to affect the GABA-mediated channel gating (i.e. which are ineffective in the absence of another ligand at the BZR) but block specifically the modulatory action of other ligands with intrinsic efficacy, are now unanimously called BZR antagonists. Reasons why the BZR is the first receptor to respond not only to full and partial agonists (with high or low positive intrinsic efficacy) but also to full and partial inverse agonists (with high and weak negative intrinsic efficacy) have been presented on several occasions (3,4,5) and shall not be repeated here. Dr. Costa (2) objects the use of the agonist-antagonists terminology with BZR mainly for two reasons. Firstly, he holds that only agonists acting at the GABA binding site should be termed agonists, and that this term should not be applied to allosteric modulators, such as BZR ligands (which, of course produce a visible effect only in the presence of a $GABA_A$ receptor agonist). There can be no doubt that intrinsic efficacy determines the action of BZR ligands in exactly the same sense as the intrinsic efficacy of $GABA_A$ receptor ligands determines their interaction with the $GABA_A$ receptor, namely by determining whether or not the ligand-receptor complex induces a conformational change with functional consequences. The agonist-antagonist terminology is of primary importance in the concept of drug-receptor interaction, while the detailed function of the receptor, i.e. whether it is a primary trigger or a secondary modulator, is of subordinate value. This by no means reduces the very important discovery and the therapeutically highly relevant fact that drugs may induce their effects by acting on a modulatory site of a transmitter receptor. Therefore, I think that for conceptual reasons the general pharmacological terms, applicable to any drug action based on the specific interaction with a receptor in biological targets, have logically to be used also for modulatory receptors, e.g. the BZR. Practical reasons to adhere to this terminology are also obvious. What would be the term for flumazenil in Dr. Costa's (2) terminology, if the agonist-antagonist concept is to be avoided? A blocker of positive and negative allosteric modulators acting at the BZR? Not very convenient, indeed. The second reason for Dr. Costa (2) to object the partial agonist concept is his statement that differing profiles of activity reflect receptor heterogeneity, which makes intrinsic efficacy superfluous. It is very important to realize that receptor heterogeneity and intrinsic efficacy are not alternatives to create and understand differences in profile. Even if one hundred different BZRs were to be found on $GABA_A$ receptors that have different affinities for various ligands, the question of intrinsic efficacy would have to be answered one hundred times, namely for every subtype individually. A pharmacologist trying to explain pharmacology without intrinsic efficacy would be in the position of an enzymologist neglecting the substrate quality of molecules binding to the catalytic site of enzymes. We have tested in our laboratories (to be published) the concept of intrinsic efficacy and partial agonism with two compounds generally believed to have each the same undiscriminative affinity for all BZR subtypes, namely the full agonist diazepam and the competitive antagonist flumazenil, by determining dose responses for various (biochemical, electrophysiological, behavioral) effects for combinations of the two compounds in differing ratios. By increasing the relative content of the antagonist in the mixture, the profile shifted from that of a full agonist to partial agonists until a pure antagonism was reached. In this way we have simulated the situation thought to underlie the action of a low-efficacy agonist, namely the simultaneous formation of effective and ineffective ligand-receptor complexes.

The way in front of us towards the detailed elucidation of the GABA$_A$-BZ receptor is long and cumbersome. Functional testing of all possible subunit combinations in expression systems and the identification of repertoires of native receptor compositions on a brain regional and cellular level will take more time than required to answer at the next Capo Boi Conference all the questions raised at the present symposium.

<u>References</u>

1. Barnard, E. and Seeburg P.H. (1988): *Adv. Biochem. Psychopharmacol.,* 45:1-18.

2. Costa, E., Berkovich, A., Wambebe, C. and Guidotti, A. (1988): *Adv. Biochem. Psychopharmacol.,* 45:367-374.

3. Haefely, W.E. (1989a): In: *Allosteric Modulation of Amino Acid Receptors: Therapeutic Implication,* edited by E.A. Barnard and E. Costa. pp. 47-69, Raven Press, New York.

4. Haefely, W.E. (1989b): In: *Antiepileptic Drugs, 3rd Edition,* edited by R.H. Levy, F.E. Dreifuss, R.H. Mattson, B. Meldrum and J.K. Perry. pp.   -   , Raven Press, New York.

5. Haefely, W. (1990): *Neurochem. Res.* (in press).

6. Hartig, P.R. (1989): *TIPS,* 10:64-69.

7. Langer, S.Z. and Arbilla, S. (1988): *Pharmacol Biochem Behav,* 29:763-766.

8. Schofield, P.R., Darlison, M.G., Fujita, N., Burt D.R., Stephenson, F.A., Rodriguez, H., Rhee L.M., Ramachandran, J., Reale, V., Glencorse, T.A., Seeburg, P.H. and Barnard, E.A.(1987): *Nature,* 328:221-227.

9. Squires, R.F., Benson, D.I., Braestrup, C., Coupet, J., Klepner, C.A., Myers, V. and Beer, B. (1979): *Pharmacol. Biochem. Behav.,* 10:825-830.

10. Verma, A., Snyder, S.H. (1989): *Ann. Rev. Pharmacol. Toxicol.,* 29:307-322.

11. Ymer, S., Schofield, P.R., Draguhn, A., Werner, P., Köhler, M. and Seeburg, P.H. (1989): *EMBO J.,* 8:1665-1670.

Subject Index

Accessory olfactory bulb, 31
Adenylate cyclase, 148–149
Adrenal mitochondrial preparations, 3
Agonist-antagonist terminology, 221–228, 232–234
AHN 086, 2
Alpidem, 61–70
  chemical structure, 62
  nigral neurons, firing, 111, 115–117
  and receptor classification, 61, 232
Alprazolam
  chronic administration, 169
  nigral neurons, firing, 111
  and TBPS binding, 91–92, 94
3-Aminopropylphosphinic acid (3-APPA), 130–131
Amygdala
  diazepine binding inhibitor products, 55
  omega receptors, 66–67
Animal studies
  chronic benzodiazepine use, 167–171
  methodological issues, 169–170
Anxiety disorders
  benzodiazepine binding inhibitory activity, 213–219
  and diazepam binding inhibitors, 202
3-APPA, 130–131
Ataxia, 80–82

Baclofen
  3-APPA comparison, 130–131
  $GABA_B$ receptors, 132
  ^{86}RB-efflux, spinal cord neurons, 147–149
Barbiturates
  α_1 and β_1 potentiation, 25–26
  nigral neurons, firing, 120
Bed nucleus, 32
Behavior, 80–82
Benzodiazepine I site
  classification, 17, 82–84, 232
  subunits, 17
Benzodiazepine II site
  classification, 17, 82–84, 232
  peptide bands, brain, 38
  regional differences, brain, 39
  subunits, 17
Benzodiazepine III site, 82–84
Benzodiazepine agonists
  chronic administration, 167–172
  conceptual issues, 221–228, 232–234
  tissue culture studies, 171–172
Benzodiazepine antagonists
  animal studies, 170
  chronic administration, 168, 170, 172–173
  conceptual issues, 221–228, 232–234
  in hepatic encephalopathy, 198–199
  tissue culture studies, 172–173
Benzodiazepine binding inhibitory activity, 213–219
Benzodiazepine inverse agonists
  animal studies, 170–171
  chronic administration, 168, 170–173

tissue culture studies, 172–173
Benzodiazepine receptor, *see* $GABA_A$ receptor
Benzodiazepines; *see also* Endogenous benzodiazepines
  chronic administration, 167–173
  in hepatic encephalopathy, 183
Beta-carbolines
  in kindled rats, 157
  nigral neurons, firing, 111–113
  receptor definition, 36
  spinal cord neurons, 143–144
  and TBPS binding, 91–94
Beta-CCM
  binding heterogeneity, 76–84
  chronic exposure, kindling, 120
  comparative pharmacologic profile, 76–82
  and ethanol, TBPS, 99–100
  nigral neurons, firing, 111–113
  rat CNS binding, 76–80
  spinal cord neurons, 143–144
  structure, 75
  and TBPS binding, 91–94
Bicuculline binding
  affinity, 37, 41
  hepatic encephalopathy, 179–180
Biculluline seizure test, 79–82
Bovine α-subunit, 44–45

CA1 cells, 132–136
CA3 cells, 133–136
Calcium, 146–149
Caudate nucleus, 66–67
Caudate putamen, 135–136
Cell line 293, 52
Cerebellum
  autoradiography, 39
  benzodiazepine ligand binding, 76–78
  diazepine binding inhibitor, 55, 205, 208
  $GABA_A$ subunits, 31–32, 39, 43–45, 84
  mRNA, subunits, 44–45
  omega receptors, 62–67
  peptide bands, 4, 43
  and receptor classification, 84
  versus spinal cord, binding, 227
Cerebral cortex
  benzodiazepine ligand binding, 76–77, 84
  $GABA_A$ subunits, 31, 43–45, 84
  $GABA_B$ binding, 136
  mRNA, subunits, 44–45
  omega receptors, 64–65, 67
  photoaffinity labeling, 43
  and receptor classification, 84
Cerebrospinal fluid, 205
CGS 8216, 182
Channel bursting activity, 223
Channel open time, 223
Chemical kindling, 153–163
  GABA function inhibitors, 153–163
  nigral cells, 120
Chick cerebral cortical neurons, 172–173

235